STOP
ANXIETY
from
STOPPING
YOU

STOP ANXIETY from STOPPING YOU

THE BREAKTHROUGH PROGRAM FOR PANIC & SOCIAL ANXIETY

DR. HELEN ODESSKY

FOREWORD BY DR. JOHN DUFFY

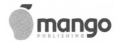

Stop Anxiety from Stopping You: The Breakthrough Program For Conquering Panic and Social Anxiety

Library of Congress Cataloging-in-Publication has been applied for.
ISBN: (paperback) 978-1-63353-546-6 (ebook) 978-1-63353-547-3

Printed in the United States of America

To Alex and Maya

TABLE OF CONTENTS

Foreword ix

Prologue. xiii

A Note about Getting the Most from this Book . xvii

PART 1: PANIC AND ANXIETY-THE BASICS

   I.   Decoding Panic and Anxiety 3

  II. The Difference between Panic and Anxiety . . . 11

**PART 2: BEGINNING YOUR PROGRAM TO
MANAGE PANIC AND ANXIETY**

  III. The U.N.L.O.C.K. System 19

  IV. Panic — The Lies 25

  V. Panic — Thinking Games. 37

  VI. Understanding Panic 55

  VII. How to Adjust Your Thinking When You Start
        to Panic 61

 VIII. Understanding Social Anxiety. 65

  IX. Social Anxiety — Negate the Lies 73

PART 3: TARGET YOUR SYMPTOMS AND DEVELOP AN ACTION PLAN

X. Action Plan – Panic: The U.N.L.O.C.K. Panic System 93

XI. Action Plan – Social Anxiety: The U.N.L.O.C.K. Social Anxiety System 103

XII. Depression and Anxiety 119

XIII. The Role of Medication 127

XIV. Troubleshooting: How to Get through Your Stuck Spots 131

PART 4: LIFELONG ANXIETY MANAGEMENT PLAN IN ACTION

XV. Maintain Your Gains for Life 139

XVI. Making Habits Stick! 173

XVII. Relapse Prevention 183

XVIII. Are You All In? 191

XIX. Anxiety Management in the Real World. . . . 197

FOREWORD

There are not many physical and emotional feelings more wildly uncomfortable than anxiety. Only anxiety sufferers truly know this for certain. For some, anxiety can feel like a background hum, a freight train of diffused fear rumbling down the tracks in the deep recesses of our mind, persistent and chronic. Others describe it as a sudden, unpredictable surge of adrenaline coursing through their veins, constricting their senses and gripping their minds with fear.

For me and many other sufferers, anxiety was a constant threat of fear and discomfort, a thief of presence and joy. At its worst, in the midst of panic, it felt embarrassing, stunningly disempowering, even life-threatening.

This was unreasonable, of course, but that is the very nature of anxiety.

An overriding anxious feeling, or outright panic, takes precedence over whatever else may be going on at any given moment in a sufferer's life. As a result, those of us who suffer, or have suffered, panic and anxiety miss out on so many of the precious moments of our lives, surrendering them to a force we know is within us, but feel we cannot control. The cycles of anxiety and panic can feel truly ominous, terrifying, and at times, hopeless. Having suffered profound anxiety myself, and treated hundreds of anxiety and panic sufferers over the past twenty years, I know this to be true.

So, we seek answers. We Google and we browse. We fill our bookshelves with the latest, greatest quick fixes. We seek therapists, psychiatrists and coaches, desperate for relief. Most of us are able to find it in these methods, but only briefly, temporarily. We learn to breathe deeply, slowly in, and slowly out. We shift our internal dialogue. We meditate and exercise. We cut caffeine from our diets.

And of course, any of these can be helpful in curbing anxiety and panic. But too often, these "solutions" are offered in isolation, the One Way to finally beat your anxiety and panic. Disappointingly, any of these alone can only be a stopgap, leaving anxiety waiting in the wings for its next opportunity.

So of course, there are countless books written on anxiety and panic, and you might be wondering why this is the one for you. I recommend this particular book, and only this book, as Dr. Odessky provides herein all of the information, tools, resources, and hope you will need to best manage your anxiety and panic. She offers success stories from her own life, and her clinical life, that will finally resonate with you. The U.N.L.O.C.K system she has developed will not only provide you with a template to refer to moment-to-moment, day-to-day, and week-to-week, but also the empowerment to truly know that you can break the cycle. In this regard, this work is wholly unique. The tips she offers are not patronizing filler, but solid tools you can put to work to mitigate your anxiety and panic right away.

Dr. Odessky has made it her life's work to alleviate the anxiety her clients and others suffer. She is tireless in this effort, and I sincerely honor this result of her work. Her knowledge, self-assuredness, and good humor will provide you immediate comfort and relief. Helen has been working for years to develop and perfect her UNLOCK program, and it works. She has come up with something revolutionary here I have never seen before: not in graduate school, not in treatment, and not in decades of reading and researching anxiety. Read this book, and you will find everything you need to beat anxiety once and for all. It's not a trick, or a quickie one-off. Instead, it is a

comprehensive, easy-to-apply system for anxiety eradi-
cation. Keep this book close. Take your time and work
through it. Trust Helen to guide you through.

It will change your life. It will free you. Finally.

Dr. John Duffy is the author of *The Available Parent: Radical
Optimism For Raising Teens and Tweens.*

PROLOGUE

Sitting in my apartment, I felt the walls slowly closing in; there was nowhere to go. This was the place I felt the safest. Now – even here – I felt on shaky ground. I was trembling, and I had what felt like a cinder block on my chest; tears welled up in my eyes, and there was nothing I could do to stop it. I felt caged, imprisoned by my emotions – with very little hope of parole. Searching to steady myself, I looked in the mirror, staring at a person I hardly recognized. This was the moment I knew that I had to do something about anxiety or it was going to consume me and run my life.

About ten years ago, shortly after being newly licensed as a clinical psychologist, anxiety hit like a tornado.

Everything in my life had been going well. I had married the man I loved, with whom I was going to build a future. The grueling days of graduate school were finally behind me. I was employed in my field of work and finally getting a steady paycheck I could actually live off. My colleagues congratulated me on passing the licensing exam, and I was getting a raise. Yes, objectively, things were going swimmingly. Inside, however, was a different story. I suddenly found myself battling severe anxiety.

I started waking up with a sense of dread. I started doubting my abilities. And worst of all, none of this made any sense to me. Now that I had finally gotten to the point where my life had become a lot less stressful and deadline-driven, now that I could finally relax a bit, how could I develop this sudden and unrelenting anxiety? I also felt as if I somehow should not have this anxiety just by virtue of being a psychologist. So I went along, putting a smile on my face and pretending that everything was okay. As you can imagine, things did not get better; I only felt more isolated, and the anxiety continued.

As I searched for a solution, I read everything I could get my hands on. I reflected on my childhood, my marriage, and my career. I engaged in journaling, examined my life choices, and consulted professionals – all with little relief. I tried every technique and searched professional literature as well as the shelves of the local bookstore. I read compulsively, but merely gaining knowledge had little to no effect on my anxiety. In retrospect, the reading became a way for me to forestall the anxiety. I was applying what I had learned, but I was quick to move on to the next strategy, hoping to hit on the Holy Grail of anxiety solutions.

Finally, I was introduced to the idea that the very battle with anxiety was the problem. I had to accept that I was anxious and live my life without being in a constant fight trying to be free of this force. This was a difficult concept to take in. I had spent a lot of time and energy fighting this enemy, and now I would have to relent. It took time and self-reflection to make peace with anxiety.

Once I did, I had to reflect on the idea that my great-on-paper life had become too comfortable. There was very little risk-taking in my life, and it was fueling my anxiety. I started making my life uncomfortable by pursuing necessary risks. I put myself in situations that made my introverted self cringe. I started pursuing activities that made me more and more uncomfortable. I left my comfortable job to go into private practice on my own. Although it did not happen overnight as I wished, I knew I was on the right track because I started feeling better. I began to recognize my former self. I was also not the same person I had been before. I had a lot more courage and I was no longer afraid of anxiety.

In retrospect, it is baffling to me that even with a doctoral degree in psychology, I did not have the resources to manage severe anxiety. It is only with a lot of research, clinical experience, and personal observations that I came up with the U.N.L.O.C.K. system to manage panic and anxiety. These days, I run a thriving private practice in Chicago specializing in anxiety treatment.

A note about getting the most from this book

If you are like many anxiety sufferers, this is probably not your first book or foray into trying to get answers and help. In fact, the very act of reading and searching for a solution is sometimes a way to manage the turmoil that anxiety causes. I get it. I have worked with hundreds of clients with anxiety and the stories I hear have motivated me to write this book. It is time to do something different. It is time to get better, and it is time to reclaim your life.

Imagine that your very good friend starts lying to you repeatedly, spreading rumors, and stealing from you. How long is that friend going to be your close confidant, someone with whom you share your innermost secrets, dreams, and hopes? How long will you continue to listen to their stories without taking them with a grain of salt or outright dismissing them? How long is it before you stop seeking their advice or inviting them to spend time with you? Probably not long, and it is probably a decision you make fairly quickly!

This is what your anxiety does day in and day out. It tells you lies: rumors about the future and half-truths about how it will affect you. It steals your time, your attention, and it is stealing the energy you have. Anxiety is a good liar; it is so good that most of us are not even aware of what is happening. All we know is that we want it to STOP.

It is natural to want to rush through and finish a book like this or just skim it for a few solutions. I invite you not to do that, so that you have time to practice the skills in this book and to really retain the information that you are learning. Slow and easy really does win the race here! I encourage you to first skim this book. After you have done so, please engage in a more thorough read the second time around. Take the time to let the information sink in thoroughly. Read and practice the exercises. Purposefully set aside time to do this for yourself – you have struggled long enough. You deserve to truly learn and master how to beat your panic and anxiety.

This book is a practical guide to managing panic and anxiety through the U.N.L.O.C.K. system. It is organized into four parts. In part one, I will guide you through the basics of understanding panic and social anxiety. In part two, I will delve deeper into the thinking processes involved and introduce the steps of the plan to manage panic and social anxiety. In part three, you will develop a plan to put the steps into action. Part four of this book will focus on maintaining gains that you make and developing lifelong habits to continue and enhance your progress with managing panic and anxiety.

Throughout the book I will guide you through a series of exercises that you can implement in your daily life. I will also encourage you to challenge some ways that you think about anxiety and to try a different approach. You will notice similarities in the approaches to panic and social anxiety treatment, with some repetition. Although seemingly redundant, there is overlap between the two entities, and looking at both serves a purpose of reinforcing key concepts. This is to be expected, and it will actually enhance your learning. As you are working your way through the program, you may notice that the skills you master will translate into you mastering situations that are outside of panic and social anxiety – when that happens to you, that is the synergy of standing up to panic and anxiety – progress often generalizes to other areas in our lives.

It has taken me a lot of professional training, research, and personal observations to finally be able to spot the lies in the information I get from anxiety. I share it in my consultation room with clients just like you who are ready to put a stop to anxiety getting in the way of what they need or want to do in their life, and I will now share it with you.

PART 1:

PANIC AND ANXIETY— THE BASICS

"It's the awareness…of how you are stuck,
that makes you recover"—Fritz Perls

CHAPTER I

Decoding Panic
and Anxiety

Before we begin working on the panic and anxiety program, it is important for you to develop a good working understanding of both concepts. We will begin by defining panic, anxiety, and fear. Next we will go through the difference between panic and anxiety. Finally, we will go over what causes anxiety and panic.

What is a Panic Attack?

"I am running. Breathless, I know there is almost no chance of survival, I know that the tornado is too close to outrun and yet I am compelled to bolt, to run away somewhere and save my life. There is no shelter, just stretches of fields — no

hope of escape. The truth is, I have never been in a situation close to a tornado — but that is what my panic attacks feel like, life or death, trying to flee desperately, only to be consumed by a force beyond my control."

"I am locked in a walk-in freezer at work, it feels like the oxygen is running out, I feel I know I am about to pass out. No one else is around — there is no hope. I wake up in a cold sweat — that time it was just a nightmare. I have never worked in food service; I have a desk job, but that is what my panic attacks feel like."

"I have been told that if a lion is going to attack you in the wild, you will not see the lion. You will only see the lion when it will be on top of you, and that is when you know you are in trouble. It is like that with my panic attacks, they just sneak up out of nowhere, and all of a sudden I know there is no escape."

"It is just like that movie where you are alone in the house, and you realize that there is a serial killer in the house with you and you are running around, out of breath, hoping to find a safe nook, and when you finally do — you are face to face! I know that there is no serial killer and that I am not in danger, but my entire body is demanding that I escape!"

Above are some examples of people describing what it feels like to have a panic attack. The danger and the push to escape are so real. Except, it does not make sense. There is no serial killer we are trying to escape. There is no mountain lion attacking us. And yet, we feel the surge of adrenalin that is coursing through our bodies with enough momentum to catapult us into the fastest sprint of our life, should we really need to save ourselves.

Irrational as we may believe it to be, our body tells us, "run for your life!" and we feel the pull, it is hard to dismiss the physical alarms. Even when there is no villain and you know that no one is chasing you. Even when there is no tornado that you are trying to outrun. This book offers you a system to overcome not only panic attacks, but also other anxiety issues, using a simple six-step process. Before we jump into the process, let's first define *panic, anxiety,* and *fear.*

Fear is an internal alarm that tells us that we are in real or perceived danger. Fear is what helps us quickly press on the brake pedal to avoid hitting a child who runs into the street. It is a built-in mechanism that helps keep us safe. Anxiety is a future-oriented response that we experience without the presence of imminent danger or threat. All of us experience some passing feelings of anxiety that are normal. For example, it is normal to feel some anxiety before a job interview or an important exam. When the anxiety becomes chronic or pervasive, or disproportionate to the stressor, it becomes an anxiety disorder. When anxiety peaks quickly and intensely, it is defined as a panic attack. You already read some examples of what it feels like to have a panic attack, below is the clinical definition.

A *Panic Attack* is defined as:
A discrete period of intense fear or discomfort in which four (or more) of the following symptoms develop abruptly and reach a peak within ten minutes. (It is entirely possible that the time it takes may feel much longer to you.)

1. Palpitations, pounding heart, or accelerated heart rate
2. Sweating, or feeling very hot
3. Trembling or shaking
4. Sensations of shortness of breath or smothering, or difficulty breathing
5. Feeling of choking
6. Chest pain or discomfort
7. Nausea or abdominal distress
8. Feeling dizzy, unsteady, lightheaded, or faint
9. Derealization (feelings of unreality), the feeling that you are in a dreamlike state
10. Depersonalization (being detached from oneself), feeling as though you are watching events happening around you from a distance
11. Fear of losing control or going crazy
12. Fear of dying

13. Paresthesias (numbness or tingling sensations) commonly felt in the fingers or toes.
14. Chills or hot flashes

Panic Physiology
The Fight or Flight Response

Our fight or flight response is hard-wired, powerful, and predictable. It is our body's way of safeguarding our survival. It pumps blood to the large muscles in the body, away from the brain, in order to ensure that we can run away from a predator in a life-threatening emergency. Our body temperature goes up, our reaction time quickens, our breathing and heart rate become faster. We are primed to react in a way that protects our survival. The flow of blood to our large muscles can make us feel lightheaded and dizzy, but it is not considered dangerous. What is happening is that you are fully alert and ready for action, should a life-threatening situation arise.

Breathing

Our breathing quickens during a panic attack. We can also feel as though we cannot get enough air or experience a choking sensation. In response, we tend to open our mouths in an effort to take deeper breaths. We may also try to correct our breathing by practicing some kind of relaxation type breathing.

I am going to go against a lot of experts who recommend different ways and types of breathing. While those techniques can be helpful in reducing your overall anxiety level, they do not help with panic. If you have ever tried to breathe your way through or out of a panic attack, it is likely that it either did nothing or that it actually escalated your panic.

Physiologically, when we think we are practicing corrective breathing, what we are actually doing is trying to take deep breaths. Most of us do this by opening our mouths to try to inhale as much air as possible. This is actually likely to increase your panic symptoms. You will probably begin hyperventilating. The very symptoms that are part of the panic profile, like dizziness, feeling faint, and lightheadedness, are actually brought on by deep, open-mouthed breathing.

Even when we are not taking deep breaths, and we are just practicing well-controlled breathing in an effort to control our panic, we are operating under an illusion. That is, we start believing that we need to take over an automatic function of our body and try to breathe intentionally. So what should you actually do when trying to breathe through a panic attack? The answer is nothing! Just close your mouth and do not interfere with your body – it knows how to breathe! It is best to let your body restore itself. If you are a fan of breathing techniques and have found them helpful, it is absolutely fine to use them, just don't use them during a panic attack. In my experience, breathing techniques can be a great way to reduce over-all stress, and they serve that purpose best when practiced regularly. I will speak to that more later on in the book.

Here's a quick tip to stop hyperventilating: The most important thing to do to stop hyperventilating during a panic attack is to close your mouth so that you do not breathe through it. Open-mouthed breathing does the opposite of what we want it to do — it will make your panic attack worse, not better.

CHAPTER II

The Difference Between Panic and Anxiety

"True happiness is… to enjoy the present without anxious dependence on the future." —*Seneca*

This is one of the most common questions I am asked in my practice: how do I know if I am having panic attacks or just anxiety attacks? A panic attack feels scary, frightening, and like you are about to lose control. It usually peaks quickly and often comes out of the blue with strong physical symptoms that typically affect breathing rate and produce a faster heartbeat.

Anxiety, by contrast, is usually a subjective feeling that may build over days or weeks, or come and go without ever turning into a panic attack, or it may come and go between panic attacks. Anxiety refers to fear in the absence of danger, and involves a future-oriented scenario. You may feel that something may go wrong: a sense of worry, dread, or a feeling of paralysis brought on by a strong sense that something (not otherwise dangerous) should be avoided. You may also experience feeling restless, keyed-up or on edge, being easily fatigued, more distractible, or have difficulty concentrating, irritability, muscle tension, gastrointestinal upset, and disruptions to your sleep. Below are two examples of what anxiety and panic feel like.

Jack came in for treatment after having several panic attacks that came on suddenly. During the panic attack, he described experiencing his heart beating very fast, feeling like he could not get enough air, and starting to feel very faint. He was also afraid that he would do something out of control, although he had not previously had any instance to suggest he actually would. All he wanted to do was to get out of the situation and to be somewhere comfortable where he could get to safety. Jack was engaged to be married to a woman he loved deeply and with whom he was excited to start a family in the near future. His current fear was that he was going to pass out during the wedding ceremony, which was going to be in a Catholic church and last over an hour. Since he would be the focus of everyone's attention, he was very worried about having a panic attack and not being able to just "slip out unnoticed."

Karen came in for a consultation due to severe anxiety she was experiencing at work. She had recently been promoted and now needed to give presentations to her department during large company meetings. Karen was terrified of public speaking. She was worried that she would do or say something that would embarrass her or cause others to think that she was not a competent professional. The night before a presentation, she could not get any sleep and noticed that she became very short with her husband and friends. Karen knew that these presentations were key to being successful in her new role, and so she endured them with great distress. Although she did not experience panic attacks, she would get sweaty palms and her voice would get shaky when she presented. This only made her more self-conscious, and she found herself over-preparing and dreading these presentations.

Both Jack and Karen (not their real names) were in quite a bit of distress when they started treatment. Jack had Panic Disorder and Karen had Social Anxiety. While only a mental health professional can provide a diagnosis, these vignettes can provide some clues into the types of symptoms you may be experiencing.

What Causes Anxiety?
We have some good ideas about what causes anxiety, and I will now share what the scientific community believes on this topic. The primary components of what contributes to the development of an anxiety disorder or panic disorder are: biology, learning, and stressors such as traumatic events.

There is a biological component to anxiety, and we know that some people are born with a more anxious temperament. This means that some people are more prone or sensitive to experiencing anxiety or responding with anxiety to a stressful situation or life event.

We also know that anxiety has a learned component. Learning theory suggests that anxiety can be acquired through learning and making associations between certain non-dangerous situations and anxious responses. This means that if we witness another person's anxious response, we may learn that that response is necessary. Children, in particular, learn about danger and safety from their surroundings. What this means is that if you had an anxious parent or caregiver, you may have inherited the predisposition to be anxious, and you may have also learned some responses that triggered anxiety in the absence of danger.

This may include behavioral and cognitive learning. Behavioral learning is learning about how to act in a certain situation. It may include learning to avoid situations that are anxiety-provoking. Cognitive learning is about how we think and assess a situation. It may include labeling certain situations as "dangerous" instead of "anxiety-provoking" or "uncomfortable." It also can prime our development of beliefs that not only is our world dangerous, but that our capacity to respond to that danger is inadequate or insufficient.

Trauma is also linked to developing anxiety. In particular, surviving or witnessing a traumatic event in childhood has been linked to changes in the brain and the likelihood of developing an anxiety disorder later in life. What we define as trauma varies, and can range from being bitten by a puppy to surviving a war. We also know that these events do not automatically result in anxiety disorders and are not destiny; they just increase the probability of a person developing an anxiety disorder.

In my clinical practice, the biggest unspoken question that I encounter is, "What did I do to get anxiety or panic?" It may not sound logical, and it is not. However, I find it is universally useful to dispel the myth that you did something to "catch" or "deserve" having panic or anxiety. To be perfectly clear, there is nothing that you did, and you are not to blame for experiencing panic or strong anxiety, PERIOD. You are only responsible for how you choose to respond to it today. As the great George Bernard Shaw said, "We are made wise not by the recollection of our past, but by the responsibility for our future."

PART 2

BEGINNING YOUR PROGRAM TO MANAGE PANIC AND ANXIETY

"Without effort and willingness to experience pain and anxiety, nobody grows, in fact nobody achieves anything worth achieving." —Erich Fromm

"The difference between try and triumph is a little 'umph.'"—Marvin Phillips

CHAPTER III.

The U.N.L.O.C.K. System

In Part One of this book we went over the basics of panic and anxiety. Now that you are familiar with both, we will go through the thinking processes involved, including panic and anxiety beliefs and the way they influence your thinking. We will also be introduced to the steps you will need to take in order to manage panic and social anxiety.

Sitting on the couch in my office, Jane looked forlorn. The anxiety she was describing seemed overwhelming to her, and she felt paralyzed to do anything about it. Her life had become a series of safe routines designed to avoid anxiety. She had changed jobs so that she could be closer to home. She barely left the house, other than to

19

go to work or run an occasional errand. Worst of all, she felt like she was perpetually in a state of dread, waiting for another anxiety attack. She looked frightened, and felt that anxiety had chained her to a life she did not want.

What Jane wanted was the key to getting better. What she needed was to unlock her power so that she could live her life, decide her direction, and exercise her freedom.

The U.N.L.O.C.K. System does just that. Through a series of exercises, I propose a framework to free yourself from the shackles of panic and anxiety and to unlock your life, your potential, and your emotional freedom. Now that you have a good understanding of both panic and anxiety, let's go over the U.N.L.O.C.K. system to begin your journey to overcoming panic and anxiety.

Step 1. Understand

The first step involves understanding anxiety and panic symptoms and their cycle. Next, we dismantle myths about panic and anxiety. Finally, we look at how we unintentionally increase our anxiety through our various attempts to control it. Understanding anxiety allows you to approach your treatment from a place of knowledge rather than fear. It includes building awareness about your symptoms and how to address them. Armed with this knowledge, you will be better able to gauge which attempts at anxiety reduction work and which make it worse. In my consultation room, often the first time that

I see relief on a client's face is when they come to understand their symptoms.

I will always remember my session with Joe; he was visibly nervous after having been referred to a therapist following two visits to the emergency room. Both visits were prompted by a feeling that he was about to have a heart attack – but after thorough physical examinations, each lasting several hours, he was medically cleared and told he was having panic attacks. Let me be clear, that is all Joe was told. He was then referred to a therapist and that is how he found himself sitting in front of me, not really sure what a panic attack was. I would love to say that Joe's story is an exception – it is not. Emergency rooms are busy places, and many people leave with no information about what their symptoms mean. As soon as I took some time to explain to Joe exactly what was happening to his body when he was having a panic attack, he became visibly relaxed. This understanding alone led him to feel much better about his situation and reduced his stress level immensely.

Step 2. Negate the Panic and Anxiety Lies

Panic and anxiety lie to you in predictable ways. It is often hard to identify this when you are in the middle of a panic attack or an anxiety attack. You will learn to identify and dispute the lies. This means that you will know that the lie is false and how to negate it.

Next, you will learn to recognize and dismiss the anxious thinking and beliefs. Once you know how to identify the panic and anxiety lies, you are free to disentangle yourself from them. Finally, you will learn how to end the argument with anxiety once and for all by refusing to argue and holding firmly onto what you know to be true.

Step 3. Leverage Your Fears

Our fears often stand in the way of confronting our anxiety. This is especially true if we believe our fears. In this book you will learn how to leverage your fears by using them to your advantage to overcome anxiety and panic. We will start by identifying your key fears. Then, we will activate them and practice them in a specific sequence so that you will be able to conquer them.

Growing up, I took martial arts. During one particular class, the instructor walked around and said, "You may not be bigger that your opponent, but if you know how, you can leverage their strength and be able to beat an opponent twice your size!" Similarly, leveraging your fears allows you to use your opponents' strength against them. This work takes time, and this is where you will need to prepare to be patient. That said, this is also where you will really start to see your progress build momentum.

Step 4. Openness: Develop an Attitude of Openness

Panic and anxiety thrive on finding dead ends, cautioning

us against remaining open to our experiences, our lives, and ultimately our selves. Anxiety breeds an attitude of wary engagement; letting you engage only when all the permutations of how something might go wrong have been run through and planned for. In the long run, this creates more stress in already stressful situations and adds tension to the most benign or even pleasant experiences. You will learn to cultivate an attitude of openness and curiosity, to remain open to the possibility of a more positive outcome.

Step 5. Compassion: Practice Self-Compassion

Panic and anxiety create a dark shroud around your life; priorities can shift from living a fulfilling life to the nearly constant management of the next anxiety symptom. A kind of fog seems to descend, and it becomes harder to keep your strengths, talents, and abilities in focus. Your goals become obscured and your direction unclear. You will learn to gain clarity with respect to life goals, valued directions, and your personal strengths. We are often our harshest judge and critic. Anxiety frequently brings with it judgment and shame. You will learn to cultivate an attitude of self-compassion so that you can remain open to attaining your goals while treating yourself kindly in the process. You will develop a habit of acknowledging your successes and giving yourself grace when you falter or make mistakes.

Step 6. Kindle: Small Changes Spark Bigger Changes

Panic and anxiety flourish in comfort. Action will be your remedy against being overwhelmed. You will learn to create momentum by making small stepwise shifts in your thinking and behavior in order to kindle your progress. Often, these cumulative little changes lead to previously unimaginable bigger shifts and sizeable changes. As Vincent Van Gogh so wisely observed, "Great things are done by a series of small things brought together."

CHAPTER IV

Panic: The Lies

"Anxiety's like a rocking chair. It gives you something to do, but it doesn't get you very far." —*Jodi Picoult*

The most urgent requests I get in my practice have to do with panic reduction. It is really something that most people are baffled by – the extreme reaction of your body, mind, and emotions can feel overwhelming and at times even cause you to question whether or not you are losing your mind. It feels like a crisis, and many people will go to their nearest hospital Emergency Room in an attempt to resolve it – only to be dismissed after hours of waiting and being told they had a panic attack.

Panic attacks can also interfere with your ability to live your life in a way you are accustomed to, as many people start to limit their everyday activities to try to avoid having a future panic attack. In our modern, western way of living, this is simply unacceptable for most people who are busier than ever and trying to get as many things done as possible. Panic attacks do not just feel like a nuisance or interference, they are often described as catastrophic to someone's life. In a culture of "busy" and "get things done" they can grind a person's life to a virtual halt. The first step towards changing this is to get past the lies and gain credible knowledge about the panic and anxiety response.

Lie Number 1: Something bad is happening!
This often sounds like the following in your head:
- **I am losing my mind or going crazy.**

The Truth: Having a panic attack is not a sign of "going crazy" or "losing your mind." It is a purely physiological reaction that can feel scary, but is not a sign of losing touch with reality.

- **I am about to die / I am very ill / There must be something physically wrong with me / I am having a heart attack, or there is something wrong with my heart or breathing.**

The Truth: These are the most common thoughts that people who struggle with panic have, and I will now show you how each one is a lie. There are certainly medical conditions that can feel like anxiety and can affect your breathing. If you are a healthy adult who gets regular medical checkups, you should mention these symptoms to your doctor and follow his or her recommendations. After a first panic attack, it is not that uncommon for someone to go to the emergency room, and it is there that physical causes are usually ruled out. If you have had a visit to the emergency room, and/or have had a physical checkup for these symptoms and have received a clean bill of health, usually your doctor will advise you to treat the anxiety or panic symptoms rather than to continue to focus on the medical side of things. If you would like a second opinion, by all means please get one. All too often, people start seeking third or fourth opinions. This, in my experience, is due to the lie that anxiety is telling you. If you have had two medical doctors give you a clean bill of health, then going back to get another opinion is how anxiety steals your time, energy, and attention. The answer at that point is to manage the anxiety or panic.

Every single person I have had the privilege of working with who suffered from anxiety or panic has told me that deep down they know whether something is anxiety or a true physical emergency or crisis. This is especially true the more panic or anxiety attacks you have had. No one can be 100% sure they are in perfect physical health, and that is how anxiety takes advantage of your vulnerability. It is probably something that you are willing to accept at most other times, since the only other option is to live in an isolation chamber hooked up to machines that will monitor you around the clock!

There is really no need for that. You know exactly what anxiety feels like. You have felt the panic before. You know exactly what the symptoms feel like in your body. And if you are feeling something that is different, that is the only time you need to seek a medical consultation.

Lie Number 2: I will pass out and embarrass or hurt myself.

The Truth: This is another common fear that I hear about in my practice. It is particularly nagging if you also experience social anxiety (the fear that any embarrassing situation will be magnified and that you will suffer a great loss of face, reputation, or even become ousted from your social or professional circle).

It is virtually impossible to pass out during a panic attack. In order to pass out, your blood pressure needs to drop. This is the opposite of what happens during a panic attack; your blood pressure rises. It is the first piece of education that I give my clients, and sadly, many have come to me after repeated consults with physicians and even mental health professionals and have not been informed of this.

The only exception that I am aware of on the entire spectrum of anxiety problems during which people can pass out are persons who have needle phobia, which is a fear of blood draws or getting medical shots or vaccinations.

Of course, anxiety tries to perpetuate this lie by demanding that you feel 100% sure this is not going to happen – which is impossible. We simply cannot rule out the possibility that someone will pass out. However, in this case, it will likely be due to a reason other than having a panic attack. I encourage you to remind yourself that you have an anxiety disorder and not a passing out disorder!

Lie Number 3: This will never end.
In your mind, this lie may sound like this: "My day or week is ruined. There we go again!" or "I will always be controlled by panic," or "I feel a little anxious now, but it is probably going to get worse."
The Truth: The truth is that even without any interference or help from us, the maximum panic response duration is about ten minutes. I understand that this in and of itself may feel like a lifetime, but this is not what most people fear. The fear is that once a panic attack starts it will bring on a long and stressful cycle of anxiety that will last a day, several days, or even weeks.

I have time and again received a raised eyebrow or a quizzical look from clients who assure me that they can have a panic attack go on for days. What is happening, once we get to the heart of the matter, is that they are cycling between lower and higher levels of anxiety without truly reaching a panic attack. (I will cover what to do about that later in the book.)

I invite you to think about your panic attack like an eye twitch; it is simply a physiological reaction. If you have ever had an eye twitch that came out of the blue, it probably felt very annoying. Typically, the more attention and energy we give it, the more stressed we become, the less likely the eye twitch is to go away. It is only when we accept it and let our body take care of it on its own that our emotional distress (feeling irritated or annoyed) is reduced and our physiology self-corrects at its own pace.

If ten minutes is still far too long for you, there are techniques you can use that will grind this cycle to a halt much faster. This will only be true once you understand and have mastered the anxiety mind game. If you believe that panic will not harm you, you will be in a position to let your body reset without interference from you. If you are still not convinced, you may have believed the following anxiety lie.

Lie Number 4: Anxiety is dangerous or "bad for me."
The Truth: Anxiety is not dangerous. Neither is panic. If you are able to get your heart rate up doing routine physical tasks like exercise, then there is absolutely nothing dangerous about your heart rate going up when you have a panic attack.

What is true is that feeling anxious and feeling excited are physiological mirror images – they are identical when it comes to your body's response. Your heart starts beating faster, and your breathing gets a little shallower, your body temperature goes up and you start feeling warmer, and you may get butterflies in your stomach. Both anxiety and excitement have this in common; it is only the mind game that is different.

Imagine for a moment the last time you felt excited about something. Your thoughts were probably something like, "I hope this goes well; this is going to be so much fun; what a great idea!" These excited thoughts were naturally positive. Now recall the last time that you felt anxious. Your thoughts probably sounded negative and maybe a bit like this: "Oh-oh! I hope nothing bad will happen; what if it does not go well? What if I mess up?" If anxiety and excitement are physiologically the same, and it is only your thoughts that are different, then changing your thoughts or how you look at and interpret your anxiety symptoms is what helps you win the mind game!

So now for the big question: is all this anxiety harmful? At the very core, anxiety tells you "yes" and that you had better follow the rules and lies that it has laid out for you. You may have grown up in a home where strong emotions were seen as dangerous, or even heard a well-meaning caregiver tell you to "save your nerves." As you may have guessed, I do not believe anxiety is dangerous. In fact, anxiety, like any other emotion, has a very important function: it is there to get your attention so that you can complete the tasks that you need in a timely manner, and to preserve your life through the "fight or flight response," which when it misfires is what we call panic.

During a panic attack, your body will go through a predictable stage of physiological activation: an area in your brain called the amygdala sends an alarm signal to your entire system. The amygdala is a complex system and is part of the limbic system, the emotional center of the brain. One of its functions is fear perception and making fear associated memories. The amygdala houses the fight or flight response, or the survival alarm in the brain. The fight or flight alarm system is so simple that it only has an "ON" and "OFF" switch. This helps with quick reaction time when faced with a bear on your hike through the woods, or with a car that slams on the brakes too quickly right in front of you. What this also means is that when this alarm system goes off, there is no input from your thinking brain as to the true degree of danger.

Like any alarm system, the one inside our brain is vulnerable to false alarms. The panic attack we experience in the absence of real life danger is not life preserving – it is simply a false alarm. The problem is that it feels identical to the signal you get during a truly dangerous situation. Like any other alarm system, our internal false alarm will sound the same every time it is triggered, even if it gets accidentally tripped. Learning to identify a panic attack as a false alarm will help you in winning the panic attack mind game.

Lie Number 5: If it makes me anxious I should avoid it.

The Truth: Repeated panic attacks can cause a lot of distress, even when you have been told they will not harm you. For this reason, many people begin to avoid situations that they associate with the onset of anxiety or panic symptoms. These situations can run the gamut of avoiding places where you have had a panic attack (like a car, if you have had a panic attack while driving) to places that you perceive as dangerous because it would be difficult to get help should you need it (like an airplane, subway or a large, crowded mall). While avoidance may make you feel better in the short run, it is guaranteed to strengthen your panic and anxiety response.

Many people force themselves to endure feared situations and do not experience a reduction in panic or anxiety. In my experience, this is typically due to the mind game and thinking patterns that can keep anxiety lingering. If the entire time you are facing a feared situation you are just hoping to get it over with, you are unlikely to get the positive anxiety-reducing value from it. You need to get back to working on your thinking game first. Otherwise, you are actually strengthening your beliefs about the dangerousness of the situation or your symptoms.

For example, if you are afraid of water, you may force yourself to go the lake and walk in ankle deep. If the entire time your thoughts are, "This is awful. I cannot wait until it is over! I hope I never have to do this again!" then no new learning is taking place. That means that you are not likely to benefit from this exercise, because what you are actually doing is cementing the learning that being around water feels awful and should be avoided.

What we want to happen during the experiential part of facing anxiety-provoking situations is to create a different type of learning. I will cover this more later in the book.

Lie Number 6: Only weak people get panic attacks.
The Truth: Having panic attacks or experiencing anxiety has nothing to do with being weak or strong. In my experience, this is a particularly difficult concept for men, but it can be for women as well. If you believe that experiencing or expressing strong emotions, any emotions, is a sign of weakness, then managing panic or anxiety will be very difficult. I offer an alternative view here. Having emotions, any and all emotions, even strong emotions, simply makes you human – and able to appreciate life fully and respond to your experience as it happens.

I frequently hear people judging themselves after a diagnosis of panic or anxiety disorder, or even just the experience of strong anxiety symptoms. Consider having hypertension, diabetes, or eczema – would you judge yourself harshly if you were diagnosed with one of these conditions? How is it different with panic or anxiety? In my view, it is not. You are simply *addressing* a real-life concern that you have as opposed to sweeping it under the rug and pretending it is not a problem. It takes strength and courage to do that!

Lie Number 7: I have to know when the next panic attack is coming.

The Truth: Panic creates a sense of urgency. It feels like you need to know for sure when the next attack is coming. Think about the rest of your life for a moment. Do you need to know the next time you will get the flu or a cold? Get stuck in a thunderstorm? Get a flat tire? You may be thinking that although you would like to have this information, it is not necessary and you can get along fine without it. Panic attacks are no different. This is a lie that panic tells you to get you to play by different rules so that it can divert your time, energy, and attention. The next time this happens, try to remind yourself that it is just not possible or necessary to have this information.

CHAPTER V

Panic-Thinking Games

"You don't have to control your thoughts. You just have to stop letting them control you."—Dan Millman

In the last chapter we covered the lies panic uses to get to you. Probably the biggest lie of all is the mind game panic draws you into. Therefore, we will now go over the thinking games that panic uses to deceive you. Panic wants you to believe that the false alarms your brain receives are really dangerous, and so it tries to engage you in several thinking games that only work out in its favor and harm you. Here are the most common thinking mistakes we make when we panic or experience strong anxiety.

1. Judgment

Problem: In the entire range of mind games that panic

and anxiety play on you, in my opinion, judgment is the most pernicious one. There are a few ways that this plays out. First, we judge ourselves for getting or having anxiety. Second, we judge ourselves for failing to get better. Third, we feel like having anxiety is shameful and we cannot talk about it, even to our closest friends and confidants. In my clinical practice, it is not uncommon for me to meet a client who has not told their spouse or close family members that they are in therapy for anxiety.

Solution: Let's end self-judgment right now. Let's put a stop to the idea that it is somehow your fault that you are anxious. It is not. Let's eradicate the idea that you should know how to deal with it – how could you? I am a trained and licensed clinical psychologist, and it took me years to crack the anxiety and panic code! How could you, without training or specialized education, possibly know how to treat anxiety and panic? You could not. Until we make anxiety education part of the health curriculum in schools and remove the stigma so that we, as a society, are able to talk more openly about it, this is an unfair expectation.

Try the following exercise to practice viewing your emotions without judgment.

Visualization Exercise to Unwind and Reset
Close your eyes and imagine a big movie screen inside

your head. In your mind's eye, go back to the start of your day, when you woke up. Going ahead in thirty-minute increments, remind yourself what you were doing, feeling, and thinking on the half hour. Do this exercise as though you are watching a movie. When we watch a movie and see a fire start, we do not run out of the movie theater as though there is real danger. Instead, we observe and pay attention without being consumed by what is on the screen. Please approach this exercise in the same way.

For example, if you woke up at 7:00 am, you may start with, "woke up, lying in bed feel sleepy, 7:30 am cooking breakfast and sipping tea, feeling relaxed, 8:00 am getting ready for work, feeling rushed," and so on. When you complete this exercise please note the absence of the words 'should' or 'should not' from it. Also, please notice how your emotions change throughout the day. Even when they are strong emotions, they all seem to pass and change.

2. Expecting the Worst

Problem: We have all been there at some time or another. A thought enters our head: "what if things get worse?" This may be during a time of stress, when we already feel like our resources have been sapped and are wondering what will happen if things gets worse. It also may happen during a time of relative calm, when you wonder, "I am okay now, but how long will it last this time? When is the next panic attack coming on?" Panic thrives on this sort of thinking – in fact, it counts on it!

Solution: The next time you have this thought, try telling yourself that it is not up to you to predict the future, and that if you did, it probably would be in the positive direction. "What if things are going to feel good for a while?" is a thought unlikely to raise anxiety!

Please remember that you are building a new habit. This means that changing your responses to anxious thoughts will feel unnatural for a while. Please expect this and practice it anyway. It takes a lot of practice to feel like a habit is becoming second nature. One way to know that it has is when it occurs to you that you have not done something you used to do in a long time. I will often have my clients notice that although they became anxious, this time they did not expect their anxiety to turn into a panic attack, as a sign of this internal change.

3. Focusing on the Negative

Problem: Panic will automatically draw your attention to the negative. In your mind, this may sound like: "This is the third day this week that I have had anxiety. I cannot believe I am still struggling! I cannot get a break, everyone could tell I started to panic at the start of my speech."

Solution: The good news is that although panic and anxiety will have you zero in on the negatives, you do not have to stay there! Zoom out and take a wider panoramic view. Ask yourself: "What is going okay? What is going well? What is going great?"

4. Ignoring the Positive

Problem: Panic thrives when it has command of all of your internal resources: your time, your attention, and your energy. When we experience anxiety or panic, it is natural to shift our resources in that direction momentarily. What you do after that initial shift determines how successful you will be at managing it. If you focus all of your energy on panic, you are likely to continue to feel worse.

Solution: If you decide to take a step back and say to yourself, "this is just part of the picture; I am also having the following positive or neutral experiences right now," and list them in your mind, you are likely to feel better. Try this exercise the next time you feel a bit of anxiety coming on:

Remove Your Internal Judge Exercise
Stop and describe everything that is in your immediate surroundings in neutral to positive terms. If you

were in the kitchen eating breakfast, it may sound something like this: "I am sitting at my wood kitchen table; it is round and I am sitting on a cushioned chair. There is a plate with a piece of toast and jam in front of me and a pot of coffee on the counter. Next to the pot of coffee is a fruit basket filled with apples and bananas. The kitchen is blue with white cabinets. The appliances are stainless steel. The floors are wood. There is a bit of sun coming through the blinds and I can see a cherry tree showing its first blossoms." Take a moment to really observe your environment and then to observe how you feel following this exercise.

If you are with people, try to describe your setting in the same manner. *"I am in a meeting with Jack and Lisa. We are sitting in a café having a business lunch. The last thing I heard Jack talking about was the new merger. Lisa was discussing some strategies to safeguard the company and Jack was offering his thoughts."* You will notice that in a few minutes your attention is pulled back into the activity of your life, rather than towards anxiety. Notice any positive effects of this exercise.

5. All or None Thinking

Problem: All or none thinking is instrumental in raising your anxiety. It works by grouping things into distinct categories, such as anxious and non-anxious, panicked and calm. Of course, in the real world, anxiety and panic do not neatly fit into such strict categories. In fact, it is not desirable to have zero anxiety – it is probably a sign that you are not fully alive.

Solution: Anxiety is not an off/on equation; it is better to think of it in terms of a range. I encourage my clients to use a scale of one through ten, one being the lowest. Try to practice rating your anxiety three times a day for an entire week using this scale. Please notice the variations throughout the day.

When we are a little anxious, it can serve to warn us that there truly is something that requires our attention: a phone call that needs to be made, a bill that needs to be paid, or an appointment that we need to get to. At higher levels of anxiety, the ones that are at the levels of panic, we may be alerted that we need to slam on our car brakes to avoid an accident, or to jump out of the way of oncoming traffic as we are crossing the street. We rarely think of the advantages of our anxiety and how we truly need it, not only to function, but also to survive in our complex world. For these reasons, it is neither attainable nor desirable to wish for its absence. What is desirable and attainable, however, is learning to respond to it in a way that does not escalate it and that is beneficial to you.

6. Catastrophizing

Problem: Catastrophizing is a process by which you take a current thought and you churn it through a series of "what-if" questions until it turns into the worst possible version of what could happen. For instance, you may think, "I feel some anxiety coming on, what if I have a panic attack when I go shopping? What if I need to get out of there quickly, without causing a commotion? I could pass out in the middle of the department store and cause an embarrassing scene. I'd better stay home today; it is going to be a miserable day."

Solution: If you notice, the initial thought just had to do with some anxiety, but once it was added onto, it became a possibly harrowing experience – with the entire day being ruined. The reality is that most of us are unable to predict the future and we do so unreliably. If you are the exception, I hope that you are getting paid handsomely for it! Try catching yourself catastrophizing when you are anxious, and ask yourself what was the initial thought or event that bothered you. It will often seem much smaller in comparison, and you will be able to downsize your reaction accordingly by responding to the initial concern or situation.

7. I Cannot Take It Anymore!

Problem: Sometimes when we struggle with something for a long time, we feel worn down and defeated. We start getting depressed and feel deflated; we feel like we cannot take another moment of struggling. This, although natural to feel, is in essence agreeing to allow panic and anxiety to run your life. This is how panic wins and you continue to feel discouraged.

Solution: Put the white flag of defeat down; do not give up the good fight! You can take it. You have lasted this far and you now have a plan to manage it, so let's start focusing on your strengths!

8. Blaming

Problem: Blaming can take several forms. We can blame ourselves, we can blame others, or we can blame a higher power. In general, I find blaming to be counterproductive.

Solution: You are not at fault for experiencing anxiety, you did not decide to have it, and you did nothing to "get" it. Blaming others offers us nowhere to go – we can only change and empower ourselves. Blaming a higher power is also counterproductive. We can choose to believe in a universal force that is punitive, or we can choose to believe in a benevolent power – the choice is yours! This brings us to the next thinking error – the "fair" universe fallacy.

9. The "Fair" Universe Fallacy

Problem: It is not a fair universe. It is not fair that you struggle with anxiety, and it is not fair that some people do not. That said, the imbalance in the universe is a philosophical problem. Our expectation that things ought to be fair is a thinking error. When we focus on it, we usually ignore the ways that the universe has been unfair in our favor.

Solution: If this is a problem for you, then try the following exercise.

Gifts From the Universe Exercise

Come up with a list of ways you have unfairly benefitted from the universe. For example, having the benefits of sight, hearing, unimpaired mobility, or excellent knowledge or ability in a certain area. Look over the list and see how you feel.

The ways that I have unfairly benefitted from the universe that are positive are:

1. _____
2. _____
3. _____
4. _____
5. _____
6. _____
7. _____

10. Mindreading

Problem: Mindreading is the act of assuming you know what other people are thinking and the inferences they are making about you. These inferences are generally skewed in the negative direction. If you are anxious or feel like you are about to have a panic attack, it may sound something like this in your mind: "Everyone will notice that I am panicked and assume I am weak or incapable of managing my emotions!" or, "She can tell my hands are trembling and she probably thinks she does not want to go on another date with me!"

Solution: In general, mindreading is wildly inaccurate. Not only are we usually way off, we forget that other people spend a large majority of their thinking time focusing on themselves and their own problems. They are also unlikely to make only negative interpretations about what other people do. If you engage in mindreading, next time remind yourself that the person is likely not thinking about you in much detail, and if they are, they are just as likely to make neutral or positive interpretations as negative.

11. Overgeneralization

Problem: Overgeneralization takes a singular event or instance in your life and applies it broadly across situations.

For example, you may say to yourself, "I had a panic attack while shopping last year. I should probably only shop with another person or avoid malls and grocery stores altogether."

Solution: The next time this happens, try saying to yourself, "This was one event, and I am not going to make broad assumptions about what will happen. I will just wait and see."

12. Personalizing

Problem: Personalizing refers to taking someone else's actions as directly related to you or a response to your behavior. For example, "He is frowning because he can tell I am nervous and not doing a good job." "She is not being friendly because she can tell I am a nervous wreck inside."

Solution: The reality is that other people's behavior is based largely on what they are experiencing and who they are. We are likely not to have enough knowledge about what is going on in their world to draw accurate conclusions. Next time this happens, try saying to yourself: "Their reaction is probably about them, and not about me."

13. "Shoulds"

Problem: "Shoulds" are the rules we play by and we are taught them in childhood. I should brush my teeth, shower daily, keep my word, right a wrong, etc. The problem comes when we try to apply these rigid rules to our emotional life. "I should not feel anxious. I should control my emotions. I should be able to stop how I feel."

Solution: Our emotional life simply does not function by such rules. I encourage you to start noticing and letting go of these emotional shoulds. They are neither necessary nor beneficial to the management of panic or anxiety. Try to maintain a measure of flexibility and self-compassion the next time you encounter an emotional "should."

14. Labeling
Problem: Labeling refers to giving yourself a negative label for experiencing anxiety, such as "loser," "weak," or even "anxious person." It sounds like this: "I am such a loser for staying home and panicking today," or "I am the most anxious person I know; I will just have to get used to feeling this way." Labeling is destructive because it berates and belittles us and diminishes our capacity for growth.

15. The grass is greener on the other side!
Problem: We have all felt it at one time or another. It just seems like other people have it easier. They are naturally able to take life in stride, to manage anxiety, or to be happier!

Solution: I find that what seems natural or effortless is

often the result of years of practicing certain habits. It is like watching a master ballerina perform; the movements are so natural that we forget they have been honed for a decade or even two! I invite you to dismiss the facade and to take what seems effortless with a grain of salt. If you struggle with this, I suggest that you adopt a mantra for what you are working on. A mantra, also called an affirmation, is a statement of positive intent that you repeat to yourself daily.

For example:

I am learning to master my anxiety better and better each day.

A life that is more peaceful and calm is on its way as I practice new skills.

I am learning to think differently in order to stop panic from stopping me.

16. Self-Pity

Problem: Struggling with anxiety and panic can be exhausting! When we are drained, our thinking can plunge into a downward spiral, and we can reach a place where we start to feel sorry for ourselves. This, in turn, can make us feel even worse and more alone than we already do. If this happens to you, it can sound like the following: "Why me? Things were okay; they were good. What did I do to deserve this? I feel so miserable!"

Solution: Self-pity is toxic and it is shortsighted. I invite you to practice self-compassion instead. Be kind to yourself, without spiraling into the negative vortex of self-pity. If you are practicing self-compassion, your thoughts sound like this: "I am really struggling with anxiety right now, but I know if I keep working on it I can get better."

17. Overthinking

Problem: We have all been there. We start thinking about something, and pretty soon we are so consumed by weighing its pros and cons, we forget why we started to think about it to begin with! Overthinking leads to delayed decisions and avoidance. Most of us think we are solving a problem when we are actually overthinking. It helps to differentiate overthinking from problem-solving.

Solution: Problem-solving involves clearly defining your situation or dilemma in the present or the very near future, generating possible solutions (a, b, c, d, etc.), prioritizing them, and then selecting which one you will act upon first. Overthinking by contrast does not define the problem clearly, is not in the present, and generates solutions that are vague and based on "what-if" scenarios. Because you cannot clearly define the problem, it is impossible to clearly outline solutions – and so it leaves you going in circles.

18. Emotional Reasoning

Problem: Emotional reasoning uses feelings as evidence of something being true. It sounds like this: "I feel bad about trying something new or anxiety-provoking, so I should not try because it is probably going to turn out badly;" or "I am so anxious, this must be a sign that something is wrong!"

Solution: The truth is, our internal wisdom is a combination of reasoning and listening to "gut feelings." Ask yourself, aside from my feelings, what other evidence do I have that this is true?

19. Holding on to the Past

Problem: It can happen so quickly. We start to reminisce and the mistakes of our past come rushing back to us, flooding our brain and evoking strong emotions of regret, anger, or sadness. It all seems so clear now – what we should have done or said. It is the benefit of hindsight that seems to make things so clear. It offers us two opportunities, one for learning about ourselves, and one for blaming ourselves.

Solution: I believe that there is everything to be gained through learning about ourselves, and nothing to be gained by engaging in blaming ourselves. I am not saying that you should not take responsibility for your actions.

Self-blame, in my opinion, is not about taking responsibility. It is about a silent ritual of reprimanding yourself without taking responsibility. It is in the learning aspect that you may decide that there is something you need to change or take responsibility for, something you wish to do differently next time. It is in the learning that we take action within ourselves, and by examining our behavior we can make decisions to act differently in the present and in the future.

What do you believe about your past? Do you believe the popular adage that "History is doomed to repeat itself"? Is it something that is destiny, or can it merely serve as a starting point for today? If you have beliefs that tie you negatively to your past, take a look at them. Your past is your past and you cannot change it. The sole value of looking at it is that you can redefine what it means in the present. If you have had a history of struggling with panic or anxiety, it is often difficult to imagine a time when it will not be so. I invite you to imagine it anyway!

Ultimately, I believe that looking at the past is only useful if it allows us to live differently in the present; to live better, more fully, more authentically today. So, if there is something that you think is related to your current anxiety, look at how those instances in the past guide your thinking and behavior today.

Ask yourself: Are you reacting today the same way you did in another situation? Does it still fit? How would you like to react today? Is there something you need to say to yourself to let go of this prior way of responding? Give yourself permission to redefine, to forgive any past mistakes, and to let go. Allow yourself to experiment with and to experience a different way of being. Notice how this feels.

CHAPTER VI

Understanding Panic

"Courage isn't absence of fear, it is the awareness that something else is important." —*Stephen R. Covey*

Your beliefs are a result of your thoughts, so check in with them, because we tend to believe what we think, and we act on what we believe. Look over the following beliefs to see how much they apply to you.

1. I am Vulnerable.

This may come as a train of thoughts related to general vulnerability, "I take things to heart so I have to be more careful," "Anxiety runs in my family so there is nothing I can do about it," or "Some people can live life and take on a calm attitude, but I am just prone to overreacting." The truth is that our beliefs are a byproduct of habits we have developed. If we say the same thing over and over to ourselves, we come to accept it as our reality.

The way we can change our habits is by adopting new ones. All we have to do is practice something different. Try changing the conversation in your mind to sound something like: "I am just as capable as anyone else at beating this anxiety or panic. Even though anxiety runs in my family, it is not destiny; I can still change the way that I respond to it. My past does not define what my future will be. If I want a calmer future, all I have to do is practice a set of anxiety management skills until they become my new habits."

2. There is only so much anxiety or upsetting emotions that I can take.

This is a common myth — that anxiety should be avoided because it will harm you and that you have to protect yourself in order to feel safe. There really is not an upper limit of what we can experience – it is just how we are built. We experience a range of emotions that run from mild to strong. All of our emotions are there for a reason, and strong emotions allow us to experience life in color – in more depth. Many of us have been taught that there are "good" and "bad" emotions. Although this belief is popular, it is untrue, and it leads us to feel shame and to judge our natural human responses. Try the following exercise.

The Emotional Acceptance Exercise

For the next twenty-four hours, whenever you experience a moderate to strong emotion, repeat this phrase:

"I feel_____ (insert emotion) and that is Okay!" Notice any effects you experience after doing this exercise.

3. I am defective / there is something wrong with me (otherwise I would have a handle on this by now).

The truth is there is nothing wrong with you just because you have anxiety or panic. This is a common problem that affects about twenty percent of people in the United States alone. Yet this is not readily discussed, and people often feel ashamed and isolated. I am here to tell you that the reasons you are having panic or anxiety are complex and are still not entirely understood. What is clear is that none of this is your fault. You did not do something wrong, nor did you "catch" anxiety or panic. It just sometimes happens, and it can feel like it takes over your life. You, my dear reader, are not at fault for getting it, and the only thing you need to focus on is how to get better!

4. I am hopeless.

There is also nothing wrong with you for not having found a solution for this increasingly common problem. I have read that people generally wait an average of seven years to seek help for anxiety. This often means that they are struggling for a long time! Beating anxiety and panic takes knowledge, skills, and practice. Just because you have not been able to find a solution previously does not mean that there is no solution or that you cannot implement it. I have seen hundreds of people get better and win their battle with panic and anxiety.

"Strength Search Exercise":

Write out a list of your strengths and accomplishments. Keep adding to this list every day for a week. If you have trouble, ask a loved one to help you get started. Notice how you feel when you read it at the end of the week.

List of My Strengths and Accomplishments:

1. _____

_____

2. _____

_____

3. _____

_____

4. _____

_____

5. _____

_____

6. _____

_____

7. _____

_____

8. _____

_____

9. _____

_____

10. _____

_____

CHAPTER VII

How to Adjust Your Thinking When You Start to Panic

"Believe you can and you're halfway there."
—*Theodore Roosevelt*

There are steps you can take when you first feel the onset of panic. First, remind yourself that your panic is uncomfortable, NOT dangerous. Second, the discomfort is temporary and will pass without your interference. Third, do the opposite of what panic wants you to do – keep the focus outward. Your thoughts will from time to time drift towards your internal sensations. Accept that it will happen and have a plan. Use the exercise about describing your space or situation in neutral terms. Focus on what you need to be doing (chores or work) or what you want to be doing (hobbies or self-care), NOT evaluating how well those things are going. Being genuinely engaged in your life versus your anxious thinking is your goal here, and the solution.

Showing Panic Who Is In Charge

In order to really overcome panic, you have to be willing to have it. As I explain to my clients with whom I experience a full range of panic symptoms in my office, once you get the hang of the mind game, you have to be willing to feel the panic in your body. For me, as it will be for you, once you get through the mind game, the panic attack becomes a non-event. Sure, you feel it, but it does not take charge; it does not ruin your day. It is like getting caught in the rain; you know it is not dangerous and the discomfort is temporary.

For these reasons, once you have worked on your thinking game, I encourage you to seek the very experiences that you find the most uncomfortable about panic. If rapid heartbeat bothers you, you can run in place until you elevate your pulse. If you dislike feeling lightheaded and dizzy, you can spin around in your chair. Once you evoke your desired symptoms, let your body restore to its pre-existing state without any interference from you. This means do not try to practice any strategy or technique to calm your anxiety or panic. Proceed with your life and notice what happens. You have to trust that your body can return to neutral by itself.

Adopt a "This Is the Way It Is!" Attitude

It is important that once you get to this step you do not engage your anxiety any more by arguing with or resisting it. You know the truth, and you do not need to convince your anxiety of anything. Arguing with panic and anxiety becomes unnecessary once you know the truth. It is another way that panic and anxiety steal your energy, time, and attention. Take on a "this is the way it is" attitude. Anxiety cannot make me pass out, and that is just the way it is. I do not know what someone else is thinking, and that is just the way it is. Practice this way of responding until it becomes second nature.

CHAPTER VIII

Understanding Social Anxiety

*"Be who you are and say what you feel, because those who
mind don't matter and those who matter don't mind."*
— *Dr. Seuss*

Mark sat in my office, perplexed. He was attractive, happily married, and had an enviable position at his company. He and his wife had a circle of friends, and he regularly played racquetball at the sports club. Recently, Mark had started to have panic attacks at work. At first, they started when Mark had to give a presentation. However, more recently he had found himself getting them out of the blue: when he was at his desk, on a conference call, or just walking to the water cooler. Mark was surprised when I suggested that he might be struggling with social anxiety.

We started talking about his life before he met his wife, Liz. Mark was generally shy around women and met Liz when they were both in college. Their freshman year, Mark was introduced to Liz by a mutual friend. Liz was a social butterfly and always had a large circle of friends. Mark quickly fit in with that circle and as a result, had a very busy social life without much effort. Later, when they got married, Liz continued to manage their social calendar. Mark often felt tired after socializing and anxious before any social event, but he assumed this was normal. He was very careful with his words and often rehearsed "small talk" topics before a party.

Things came to a head when Mark was promoted to a position where he had to take impromptu meetings and deliver company-wide reports. Without his preparation, Mark felt panicked, sure that he was going to say something foolish and become the laughing stock of the company. He went to work in a state of dread and frequently experienced panic attacks prior to starting therapy.

Mark's problem is a common problem. In the United States, forty million adults struggle with an anxiety disorder, fifteen million adults struggle with social anxiety, and six million face panic disorder (adaa.org, accessed July 23, 2016). It is common for social anxiety to co-occur with panic disorder, and people frequently think it is panic that is the problem. The real issue only comes out after someone fully explains their experience and symptoms in my consultation room. Usually if you have social anxiety, you are also very worried about the social consequences of having panic attacks or any visible signs of anxiety. If you have social anxiety, you may be extremely uncomfortable in social situations and try to avoid them. You may feel intense anxiety about being judged by others and live in fear of doing or saying something shameful or embarrassing. When you do participate socially, it may feel as though there is a spotlight shining on you and all your mistakes will become not only visible, but also magnified. Because these situations are so difficult for you, you may not be able to do the things that you would like, such as dating and certain social, school, or work activities. A subset of people with social anxiety experience it only in performance situations, such as public speaking or performing on stage or in front of people.

> Janet came in for a consultation due to experiencing frequent panic attacks. She described that they usually occurred when she was invited to a party. She would notice the anxiety building prior to the party and the day of. She would dread having to go

for fear of embarrassing herself. She felt like if she went with other people, they would notice if she had to leave early (due to panic), and so she often went by herself and did not enjoy it. Sometimes she avoided the parties altogether, fearing that her symptoms might get so bad that they would be noticed. When she did go, she felt like there was a big spotlight on her and that any social error that she made was magnified.

Janet's experience is common among people who struggle with anxiety. Let's take a look at the formal clinical definition of social anxiety as defined by the Diagnostic and Statistical Manual V, published by the American Psychiatric Association. The current definition of social anxiety according to *DSM V* is:

A. A persistent fear of one or more social or performance situations in which the person is exposed to unfamiliar people or to possible scrutiny by others. The individual fears that he or she will act (or show anxiety symptoms) in a way that will be embarrassing and humiliating.

B. Exposure to the feared situation almost invariably provokes anxiety, which may take the form of a situationally bound or situationally pre-disposed panic attack.

C. The person recognizes that this fear is unreasonable or excessive.

D. The feared situations are avoided, or else are endured with intense anxiety and distress.

E. The avoidance, anxious anticipation, or distress in the feared social or performance situation(s) interferes significantly with the person's normal routine, occupational (academic) functioning, or social activities or relationships, or there is marked distress about having the phobia.

F. The fear, anxiety, or avoidance is persistent, typically lasting 6 or more months.

G. The fear or avoidance is not due to direct physiological effects of a substance (e.g., drugs, medications) or a general medical condition not better accounted for by another mental disorder...

Copyright 2013, The American Psychiatric Association

At the heart of it, social anxiety is about the fear of judgment and embarrassment. It is understandable – most of us do not want to be ousted from our social circle. From an evolutionary perspective this makes sense – you were much more likely to survive if you were with your tribe;

you would have protection and access to shared resources. People struggling with social anxiety often would like to have control over how they are perceived by others and have fairly strict rules about what constitutes acceptable behavior in a social situation. As a result, if you have social anxiety, you may have adopted the philosophy of "niceness" and politeness to a fault. This belief is often recognized by the person struggling with social anxiety as unreasonable or excessive, however, it is usually so powerful that it becomes the guiding force in making decisions about whether or not to engage in feared activities.

In order to overcome social anxiety, it is necessary to first understand the social anxiety mind game and to correct the anxiety lies. Second, it is important to challenge any thinking errors and beliefs that drive social anxiety. Third, it is time to look at any behaviors that you are avoiding or enduring with intense anxiety and to start systematically engaging in those behaviors again until they no longer produce the same effect.

Every person who experiences social anxiety feels it a bit differently. Below is a partial list of situations that may produce social anxiety. Please read it over and see which may apply to you:

- Eating or drinking in public

- Flirting

- Trying to ask someone out on a date

- Speaking in public

- Taking part in a performance, such as being in a play

- Singing on stage or participating in karaoke

- Giving a toast at a wedding

- Speaking to someone in authority

- Returning a purchase to a store

- Attending a party or social gathering

- Hosting a party or social gathering

- Urinating in a public bathroom

- Speaking up in class or at work

- Talking with someone you do not know well or who is a stranger

- Entering a room after the meeting or a party has already started

- Being observed while you work

- Calling someone who you do not know well or who is a stranger

- Dancing in public

- Making eye contact with someone you do not know well

- Being the center of attention

- Talking with or being introduced to people of authority

- Being teased or criticized

Please write down any additional situations not covered by this list that produce social anxiety for you:

_____

_____

_____

_____

_____

_____

_____

_____

_____

_____

_____

_____

CHAPTER IX

Social Anxiety — The Lies

"You have brains in your head you have feet in your shoes. You can steer yourself any direction you choose. You're on your own. And you know what you know. And YOU are the one who'll decide where to go." —Dr. Seuss

Your social anxiety lies to you in the following ways:

Lie Number 1: People can tell I am anxious and they will judge me harshly for it.

The truth is, most of the time people are unaware of your internal state. They are also fairly focused on themselves, and so they are probably thinking about their own problems and feelings. Sometimes you may have overt signs of anxiety: you turn bright red, stammer, or you sweat profusely. I would say that most people are still not going to jump to the conclusion that you are anxious. For example, they may think you are feeling warm, ate something spicy, or are getting sick.

Let's assume that someone does notice your anxiety. What would that mean? Your social anxiety tells you that they will think less of you. The truth is they probably will relate to you or at the very least empathize. It is our imperfections that make us human, relatable, and able to connect.

Think about someone you know who is so together that they appear "perfect." How relatable do you find that person? How much do you like them and want to be emotionally close to them? The answer is probably not much – they are too difficult to relate to! Now think for a moment of your closest friends whose flaws you are well aware of and have come to accept. How much do those flaws affect your view of them as a great person and a good friend?

The good news here is that your anxiety is personal and largely noticeable only to you. On the rare occasion that people may notice, I would venture to say it simply makes you more endearing and more likable!

Lie Number 2: There is always a right and a wrong way to act in a social situation.

If you noticed the all-or-nothing thinking error here, way to go! This is a false dichotomy. Social situations are complex and nuanced – there is no one right way, and searching for one is fruitless. In fact, each culture and sub-culture has many variations on what is considered appropriate social behavior. We all do the best we can socially, and if we make a mistake, all we can do is to learn from it and move on.

Lie Number 3: I have to try to control other people's opinions of me.

Thousands of years ago, the famed Greek philosopher Plato said: "We cannot control our reputation." It is still true today. Let's give up this illusion of control as quickly as we can by focusing on what we truly can do – live with integrity by acting on our values and keeping our word. Let go of the rest.

Some people are in the business of reputation management and witness the engineering of perception in their daily work lives, so it is hard to believe that we cannot control it. I hold it to be true that while our actions and words can influence our reputation, they cannot control it entirely. People are free to make up their own minds, regardless of how much we may not want it to happen.

Lie Number 4: Other people are very critical of mistakes.

Your social anxiety is telling you that other people will be harsh and critical of you if you make a mistake.

Bob was brutally teased in middle school. He was smaller in stature than other kids his age and had a stutter. This made him extremely cautious of public speaking. Though he outgrew his stuttering a few years later, he still felt that he might stumble over his words and be teased and embarrassed. As an adult, he became very nervous at any speaking opportunity. As a result, he avoided speaking up at work, even when he thought it would benefit him professionally.

Bob's story is not uncommon. If you have ever been the object of teasing or bullying as a child, the ill effects can often stay with you into adulthood. Kids can be outright brutal in their teasing. In part, this is due to the fact that their ability for empathy is still developing. Adults tend to be much more compassionate and tolerant of differences. If this is an issue for you, please consider how you would respond if someone else made a mistake in public. Would you try to say something to highlight their embarrassment or mistake, or would you respond with compassion? If you answered that you would respond with compassion, isn't it likely that others would respond in kind?

Thinking Errors

If you struggle with social anxiety, you are probably making some or most of the following thinking errors. Some of these thinking errors are similar to the panic thinking errors that we went through earlier, and you will notice some overlap and similarities.

- **Personalizing**

  Problem: Assuming that someone's negative behavior is in direct response to you.

  Solution: Other people's behavior usually has a lot to do with them; who they are, what is happening in their life, how much sleep they got the night before, and so on.

- **Mindreading**

  Problem: Assuming you know what someone is going to think about you.

  Solution: We do not know what someone else is thinking; it is better to focus on being kind in our thoughts towards ourselves.

- **Labeling**

  Problem: You refer to yourself with names, like "I am a loser," or "I am boring," or "I am just not good at being social."

  Solution: We know that labeling is going to make you feel lousy and increase your anxiety. You are better off practicing compassionate self-talk.

- **All-or-Nothing Thinking**

  Problem: Looking at things in categorical or diametrically opposed terms. For example, "I am either anxious or everything is fine." "I am either well regarded or people think I am a social failure."

  Solution: Most situations in life are dimensional. Anxiety is something that runs from mild to medium to high in level. Embarrassment can also run mild to medium to high. When you notice that you are focusing on extremes, try to remind yourself to look for a middle ground.

- **Fortune Telling**

  Problem: Assuming you will know how the situation will turn out. "I should skip the party because I will be miserable and have a terrible time," or "I had better come up with an excuse not to do that presentation, because if I do it, everyone will know how incompetent I am."

  Solution: Keep your focus on the situation at hand, by looking at the present moment and what you need to be doing right now.

- **Discounting the Positive**

  Problem: You focus only on the negative aspects of

the situation, and ignore or minimize what went well. *Solution*: Anxiety will produce the negative feelings and thoughts automatically. All you need to do is to supplement the positives to balance out the picture.

• **Focusing on the Negative**
Problem: You focus only on the negative aspects of the experience and keep replaying them in your mind (also called "the postmortem"), or keep trying to rewrite a negative event in the past.

Solution: Instead, look at what is going well or what went well.

• **Catastrophizing**
Problem: You focus on the worst possible outcome when you take the initial scenario through a series of "what if" questions.

Solution: Focus on the present moment and the situation you have to deal with at this moment. Go back to the original problem, rather than solving hypothetical ones.

• **Good Things Happen to Good People**
Problem: You assume that by acting flawlessly in

social situations you are assured of social success and can avoid having any social mishaps or embarrassment. You adopt an attitude of politeness even when it does not benefit you.

Solution: There is not always a way to be "nice" or "polite." Sometimes you have to be assertive and set limits, address an uncomfortable issue, or simply walk away. There are no perfect social interactions, and even when a situation does not go flawlessly, people usually move on quickly.

Social Anxiety Beliefs

Please look over the following social anxiety beliefs to see if they apply to you to any degree.

1. I Am Not Likeable.

Problem: Social anxiety can make us question our very likeability and desirability as a social companion. We may start to wonder if we are simply less likable than other people and therefore have more difficulty in social interactions. This is a common belief, and so it is important to examine.

Solution: Let's look at some people in the world who had social success and were not very likeable. Adolf Hitler was a great orator as well as an atrocious human being who was responsible for mass genocide. Charles Manson was a convicted mass murderer, and he was also charming and very successful socially, and attracted many women. My point is, let's really take your likeability out of it. In my experience, I have not met a single person with social anxiety who I thought had a "likeability" issue. Let's just assume that you are likeable. This does not mean that you will be liked by everyone. We cannot control that. Some people simply will not like you, and that is okay. Really, not everyone will or has to like you. This is not the problem you need to solve. You need to be okay with people not liking you some of the time for reasons unknown to you.

2. I am not Worthy.

Problem: Perhaps, underneath, you wonder if you are good enough or "worthy" of good social connections or experiences.

Solution: "Affiliation" or being close to other humans is a basic human need. There is nothing you need to do to earn it; you are already deserving of it. If you do not feel this way, please ask yourself, "What makes me not worthy?" A lot of the time, the answer is "nothing" and it frees you to move on. Sometimes the answer reveals an insecurity you have about yourself and your social desirability: "I am not very attractive," "I am not very eloquent," or "I do not have a great sense of humor." At other times there is just a vague sense of not being good enough. No matter what your personal answer is, it is very likely that you are applying perfectionistic standards here. No one has flawless beauty, 100% perfect elocution, or unfailing humor. Beauty queens have their photos airbrushed to remove flaws, professional speakers fumble and make errors, and great comedians make bad jokes from time to time. Shift the focus to your strengths and you will start discovering what you bring to the table, rather than what you lack.

3. I am Helpless.

Problem: If you struggle with social anxiety, it is not uncommon to start over-relying on very social friends or family members in order to feel more comfortable. It can become a crutch to only engage in social situations with people with whom you feel "safe." It limits you socially, and it reinforces the belief that you just cannot do it yourself.

Solution: I encourage you to reduce and then eliminate these crutches as soon as you are able to.

Engage in your feared behaviors without "safety people" or "safety objects." It is just a matter of practice before it gets easier.

Write down any negative social anxiety beliefs that may apply to you, including those that may not have been listed above:

_____

_____

_____

_____

_____

_____

_____

_____

_____

_____

_____

4. There's A Right Way to Act in Every Situation

Problem: When you struggle with social anxiety it feels like there is an exact way to act in every situation, and when we fail to do so, or believe that there is a strong chance that we will not be able to do so, our anxiety spikes. To make matters worse, we sometimes doubt that we can figure out what that exact right way to act is, and we may suffer mercilessly trying to bridge the gap or avoid the situation altogether.

Solution: I would encourage you to start noticing when others who you admire make social mistakes or "break" the social code slightly. What are the consequences? How do they handle it? Is it possible that it largely goes unnoticed, or is quickly dismissed?

Safety Behaviors

We all do things to make ourselves more comfortable if we can. In the case of social anxiety, this can turn into a ritual that silently promotes and exacerbates anxiety. For example, you may always have a glass of wine before you feel okay socializing. It is not that you have a problem with alcohol; you have just developed a ritual and you now feel handicapped without it. Some examples of safety behaviors are:

- Always needing to be accompanied by people you know well in social situations – without an otherwise obvious necessity to do so.

- Always having a drink or two at a party or social gathering before you feel relaxed enough to socialize.

- Always engaging in an activity at a social gathering with the purpose of avoiding socializing, such as regularly cleaning up, helping the host with serving food, or any other activity that gets you out of just being a guest.

- Feeling the need to carry around an object with you that you feel safe with: a rabbit's foot, your lucky rock, or even your anxiety medication that you usually do not need.

- Asking for reassurance repeatedly (e.g. about appropriate social behavior, what you wear, how you come across, etc.)

- Over preparing for a presentation or performance.

- Having to repeat a behavior before you feel it is okay to be out socially: This can be excessive grooming or spending a very long time to apply makeup, do your hair, or select just the right clothing. Having to look in the mirror very carefully, having to recite a prayer or an encouraging statement, or feeling the need to read certain pages in your anxiety book in order to feel "okay" to socialize.

Safety behaviors are a form of avoidance. They block

you from fully feeling your anxiety and also from the benefit of watching your anxiety diminish on its own. For this reason, it is important to work on eliminating any and all safety behaviors from your repertoire. Start by making a list of all the safety behaviors you practice and ranking them from easiest to toughest to give up. Then, start by eliminating the easiest one, and then move toward the more difficult ones. If this proves challenging, you may wish to seek help from a friend who can hold you accountable or retain the services of a licensed therapist who specializes in treating anxiety.

Think of any safety behaviors that you currently have and write them down below:

_____

_____

_____

_____

_____

_____

_____

_____

_____

_____

_____

_____

Social Anxiety Key Fears — Your *Personal So What*

Think about your key fears. The clues often lie in activities that you avoid or endure with a lot of anxiety. It is often helpful to ask yourself what would happen if what you imagine – the worst of it – actually happens? I call this your *personal so what*. It works like this:

For example: If you are afraid of public speaking, ask yourself:

Q: What would happen if I messed up during a presentation?
A: I would be laughed at.

Q: So what?
A: People would think I am not very smart.

Q: So what?
A: So I would not get promoted.

Q: So what?
A: So I am not going to get very far in my career.

Q: So what?
A: I will be a failure.

In the above scenario, that's the key fear – making an error and being seen as a failure.

Below is a list of social anxiety key fears:

- Making a mistake in public and being seen as a failure or incompetent

- Judgment, being seen as inferior or not good enough

- Doing something that elicits laughter or ridicule from others/embarrassment; being seen as unlike-able or unlovable

Think about your *personal so what* and write down your key fears:

_____

_____

_____

_____

_____

_____

_____

_____

_____

_____

_____

_____

Avoiding Positive Attention

Thus far, we have been focusing on the role of social anxiety in avoiding negative or undesirable social consequences: the fear of being ridiculed, judged or embarrassed. It is also important to look at how you handle positive attention if you have social anxiety. Positive attention is attention that you receive when something is going right, such as a compliment, praise, or formal recognition during an award ceremony.

If you are like most people with social anxiety, you are also avoiding positive attention. Usually this is done in an effort to avoid judgment or embarrassment should you unintentionally do something wrong. Yes, if you have social anxiety, any attention seems to be undesirable. This can be quite problematic, as we are socially mandated to draw attention to ourselves some of the time. Birthday celebrations, graduations, and certain work functions are some examples of those situations where you are expected to receive positive attention.

Start by making a list of the situations that you avoid that can garner positive attention. Next, rank your list from easiest to more difficult items and start practicing with the easier items first, moving to the more challenging ones as you complete them.

Think about situations that you are avoiding where you may receive positive attention and write them down:

_____

_____

_____

_____

_____

_____

_____

_____

_____

_____

_____

_____

_____

_____

PART 3

TARGET YOUR SYMPTOMS AND DEVELOP AN ACTION PLAN

"Inaction breeds doubt and fear. Action breeds confidence and courage. If you want to conquer fear, do not sit home and think about it. Go out and get busy."
—Dale Carnegie

CHAPTER X

Action Plan - Panic: The U.N.L.O.C.K. Panic System

Thus far, we have discussed how to manage the thinking and beliefs that are involved in managing panic and anxiety. This next part of the book will focus on developing a specific action plan for both panic and social anxiety. If you are noticing overlap and repetition, that is because the treatments for both have some similarities, and you have probably mastered some of these concepts by now – which is good news. The key part of this section is focused on action steps. I suggest that you take your time here, develop your individualized action plan, and implement it. If you experience difficulties or snags, there is also a chapter on how to get through your stuck spots.

Your action plan for panic involves the following steps using the acronym U.N.L.O.C.K. to help you remember:

1. **U**nderstand. Understand the truth about panic symptoms and their cycle, and be able to identify the lies that panic is telling you.

2. **N**egate. Negate and dismiss panic thinking errors. Recognize and dispute negative beliefs that fuel panic.

3. **L**everage. Leverage your Fears (Feared Panic Symptoms) and practice them. Practicing your feared panic symptoms until you are no longer afraid of them will give you leverage to overcome them.

4. **O**penness. Develop an attitude of openness to the idea that you will develop a very different relationship with panic and the way that it influences your life. Develop an attitude that things may go better than you expect.

5. **C**ompassion. Develop self-compassion and practice it.

6. **K**indle. Kindle bigger changes by starting with small steps. Begin by facing your less-feared symptoms and situations first to build the momentum to move on to more-feared symptoms and situations.

Step 1: Understand Panic

Review the truth about panic earlier in this book. Write down any lies that panic is telling you and dispute them below.

Example: Panic is telling me I will pass out, even though it is counter to the true physiology of my body.

_____

_____

_____

_____

_____

_____

_____

_____

Step 2: Negate the Lies

Write down the thinking errors that happen when you experience panic or that are likely to lead to more panic symptoms:

1. _____

2. _____

3. _____

4. _____

5. _____

Write down any negative or unhelpful beliefs that are activated and why they are false:

1. _____
   _____
   _____
   _____
   _____

2. _____
   _____
   _____
   _____
   _____

3. _____
   _____
   _____
   _____
   _____

Step 3: Leverage Your Fears

It is now time to leverage your fears. Remember that even if you feel your opponent is stronger than you are, you can leverage their strength against them and win! In the case of panic, we will use bringing on panic symptoms rather than trying to suppress them to create exposures that lead a to win. We will use the symptoms to help your treatment, rather than trying to run away from or fight them. This is how we take away its power, by directing it towards the goals that serve YOU.

Write down the symptoms that bother you the most during a panic attack (the scariest ones):

For example: Fast breathing, dizziness, nausea, tingling in hands, and rapid heartbeat.

List of my feared symptoms:

_____

_____

_____

_____

_____

Next, write down a list of activities that you will practice that will help bring on those sensations.

List of feared symptoms and activities I will practice.

For example:
- Rapid heartbeat – sprint or run in place vigorously for 60 seconds to get my heart rate up
- Feeling dizzy – spin in a chair
- Feeling faint – breathe through a small straw

1. _____
2. _____
3. _____
4. _____
5. _____
6. _____
7. _____
8. _____
9. _____
10. _____

After your practice, review the list of activities and any beliefs that sabotage your efforts or progress. Write them down below:

_____
_____
_____
_____
_____
_____
_____
_____
_____
_____
_____

Practice until you are no longer afraid of your symptoms. This type of practice is called exposure, because you are exposing yourself to, or facing, your feared symptoms. During this practice do not try to reduce your anxiety in any way, either through any thinking methods or breathing activities or other relaxation behaviors. Please note any safety behaviors. As you recall, safety behaviors are any actions or rules that you follow that reduce your panic or anxiety sensations. Safety behaviors will interfere with your exposures. It is usually preferable to attempt an easier exposure without the use of a safety behavior, rather than trying a more difficult exposure while engaging in safety behaviors. Trust, that if you have done the work on the panic thinking game prior to this exercise, your anxiety will reduce on its own without help from you – just keep practicing.

Step 4: Openness: Be Open to the Possibility of Change

Write down what you will feel, think, and do when you are no longer afraid of your panic symptoms. List a more positive outcome than you typically expect. (For example, if you typically think: "this will never work," you can change it to: "I cannot predict the future, and there is a chance that this will work out and I may be further along than before I tried this.") Go ahead and write down a statement that reflects openness towards a different, more positive outcome below:

_____

_____

_____

_____

_____

_____

_____

_____

_____

_____

_____

Step 5: Compassion

When change is incremental and you are focusing on the long game, it is important to remain compassionate with yourself when your practice sometimes goes imperfectly or you make mistakes. This means speaking to yourself in a way you would speak with a good friend or a young child, gently and without harshness.

(For example, "I am learning a series of skills and I will make mistakes along the way. That just means that I am human.") *Please write down some compassionate ways you can respond to yourself when you feel unhappy with yourself or your progress:*

_____

_____

_____

_____

_____

_____

_____

_____

_____

_____

_____

Step 6: Kindle — Small Changes Spark Bigger Changes

Write down a list of activities that you have been avoiding or enduring with a lot of distress due to the fear of experiencing panic symptoms. Next, rank them from easiest to more challenging. Start with the easiest one, moving towards the more challenging items:

1. _____
2. _____
3. _____
4. _____
5. _____
6. _____
7. _____
8. _____
9. _____
10. _____

Practice until these activities no longer produce anxiety and you no longer fear engaging in them.

CHAPTER XI

Action Plan-
Social Anxiety:
The U.N.L.O.C.K.
Social Anxiety System

"To learn and not to do is really not to learn. To know and not to do is really not to know." —Stephen R. Covey

Here is your U.N.L.O.C.K. action plan to beat social anxiety:

1. **Understand.** Understand the truth about social anxiety and be able to identify the lies that social anxiety is telling you.

2. **Negate.** Negate and dismiss social anxiety thinking errors. Recognize and dispute negative beliefs that fuel social anxiety.

3. **Leverage.** Leverage your social anxiety fears by practicing them until you are no longer afraid of

them. Identify your *personal so what*. Develop a list of behavioral exposures to activate your key fears, rank them, and engage in them starting from the easier to the more challenging.

4. **O**penness. Develop an attitude of openness to the idea that you will develop a very different relationship with social anxiety and the way that it influences your life. Be open to a more positive outcome than your social anxiety suggests is likely.

5. **C**ompassion. Develop self-compassion and practice it.

6. **K**indle. Kindle bigger changes by starting with small steps. Begin by facing less-feared situations and move on to situations that elicit greater fear in order to create momentum and create bigger changes.

Step 1. Understand Social Anxiety

Review the lies social anxiety is telling you that were covered earlier in this book. Write down any lies that social anxiety is telling you and dispute them below.

Example: Social anxiety is telling me that everyone is focusing their attention on my behavior, even though people are usually busy focusing on their own lives and their own problems.

_____

_____

_____

_____

_____

_____

_____

_____

_____

_____

Step 2: Negate the Social Anxiety Thinking Errors and Negative Beliefs

Write down the thinking errors that happen when you experience social anxiety or that are likely to lead to more social anxiety symptoms:

1. _____

2. _____

3. _____

4. _____

5. _____

Write down any negative or unhelpful beliefs that are activated for you by social anxiety and why they are false:

1. _____

_____

2. _____

3. _____

3. Leverage Your Key Fears

Write down your key fears.

Example: Making a mistake, judgment from others, doing something that other people might laugh at or ridicule.

1. _____
2. _____
3. _____

Write down a list of activities that activate the key fears for your behavioral exposures. During your practice, do not laugh off your embarrassment or act in any way to suggest that your actions are a joke.

Sample list of activities that activate the fear of making a mistake:

1. Ask for change or buy something with cash at a store and challenge whether the amount you received was correct, count the change slowly, and recognize your mistake.

2. Press the wrong elevator button (or several) in an elevator with other people that you do not know. The best way to do this is to wait in the lobby of a tall building until a few people walk in. Next, wait for them to press the button of the floor to their destination. Once they are finished, make sure to press a button (or several) that is below what has already been selected. Your goal is to have your behavior stick out and to, albeit minimally, affect the other passengers.

3. Deliberately mispronounce something, like a common drink at your local coffee shop. Make this obvious and do not laugh.

Sample list of activities that activate the fear of judgment:

1. Make a visit to a high-end store or boutique wearing simple clothing, such as a tee shirt and pajama pants or sweatpants. Ask the salesperson to show you one of the more expensive items they sell.

2. "Accidentally" knock down a few non-fragile items from a display stand at the store (such as scarves or hats). Make your error noticeable as you are picking the items back up.

3. "Accidentally" drop a plastic bottle or cup full of water. Mop up the spill yourself or get an

employee to notice that you need help.

Sample list of activities that activate the fear of being laughed at or ridiculed:

1. Go to a drugstore and pick out several boxes of feminine hygiene products or contraceptives. Take them to the cash register and ask how much they cost. After you get your answer, politely say, "I'm afraid that's just too much for me," and walk out.

2. Go to a department store and ask for an item that does not exist or is not sold at the store that would be embarrassing. For example: extra small condoms, a vibrator, or a medicine that can take away cellulite, etc.

3. Tuck a strip of clean toilet paper so that it sticks out of the back of your jeans or pants. Make sure the toilet paper is visible, not covered by your jacket or outer layer. Take a ten-minute walk on a busy pedestrian street. If someone notices and comes up to tell you about it, say thank you and move on.

My List of Activities that activate key fears:

1. _____

2. _____

3. _____

4. _____
5. _____
6. _____
7. _____

Step 4. Openness

Develop an attitude of openness to the idea that you will develop a very different relationship with social anxiety and the way that it influences your life.

I will ask that you imagine a very different way of being. As a first step, I'd like you to become open to the idea that something that scares you very much may not be all that frightening once you do it. Next I will ask you to be open to the idea that it may go better than you imagined it. Then I will ask you to imagine a time when you will feel excited by, rather than afraid of, your social anxiety fears. Finally, I invite you to be open to mistake making as an opportunity to discover something new.

Step 5. Compassion

Develop Self-Compassion and Practice It.

I am asking you to do things that up until now you have probably been avoiding or engaging in with a lot of anxiety. Sometimes when you make changes it will feel very easy. At other times it will feel slow, with progress nowhere in sight. During those times, you may find that it feels as though you are walking in water, at a pace much slower than you are used to moving. Understand that progress varies and allow yourself to move at your own pace. Change can sometimes be difficult, and you need to give yourself a break and practice a little self-compassion when things don't progress as quickly as you think they should.

Step 6. Kindle. Small Changes Spark Bigger Changes.

Write down the situations that trigger the most social anxiety for you.

For example: Public speaking, going out on a date, going to a party, flirting, or calling someone you do not know very well.

List of My Feared Situations / Situations that Create Significant Discomfort.

1. _____
2. _____
3. _____
4. _____
5. _____
6. _____
7. _____
8. _____
9. _____
10. _____

Write down the activities you will engage in to practice being in feared situations, ranking them from lowest to highest (rate them on a scale of 1-10, with 1 being the lowest in anxiety). Start your practice with activities that rank at a difficulty level of 3-4. If you are not a fan of using numbers, you can rate them "very easy," "easy," "moderate," "challenging," and "very challenging." Start with activities in the "easy" range.

Next, create a "willingness" chart, ranking how willing you are to do each of the feared activities in order. You are making a willingness list in order to tap into what you value. If social anxiety is showing up in multiple situations for you, you can often be guided by what you would love to change the most. For example, if social anxiety has been a huge barrier to romantic relationships, your desire to start dating may make you more willing to prioritize that area for exposures. On the other hand, if you are facing difficulties in your career due to fear of public speaking, this may make you more willing to tackle that area of your life.

My willingness hierarchy (1-10, with 1 being the task you are willing to do first):

1. _____
2. _____
3. _____
4. _____
5. _____

6. _____

7. _____

8. _____

9. _____

10. _____

Review this list following each activity to see if you need to update the order, as you may be spurred on by your success and develop increased willingness to do activities that you were previously very hesitant to engage in.

Sample list of social anxiety feared activities for public speaking:

Ranking of 1: Practicing my speech in front of a friend.

Ranking of 2: Speaking for five minutes at a group meeting at work with five coworkers and my supervisor present.

Ranking of 3: Giving a toast at my father's 60th birthday party.

Ranking of 4: Taking the lead at a teleconference meeting at work; speaking for 30 minutes.

Ranking of 5: Reading a poem I wrote in front of an audience at a neighborhood open mic night.

Ranking of 6: Attending a speaking organization meeting and introducing myself.

Ranking of 7: Giving a presentation at work for an hour.

Ranking of 8: Presenting a project proposal at a homeowner's association meeting.

Ranking of 9: Presenting at a business association meeting.

Ranking of 10: Giving a speech at a speaking organization meeting in front of 50 people.

Next, create a list of your personal rank ordered list of feared activities.

Ranked list of feared activities I will practice with the corresponding level of fear or anxiety:

Activity	Willingness Rank
_____	_____
_____	_____
_____	_____
_____	_____
_____	_____
_____	_____
_____	_____
_____	_____
_____	_____
_____	_____

After your practice, review the list of activities and any beliefs that sabotage your efforts or progress. *Write them down below:*

_____

_____

_____

_____

_____

_____

_____

_____

_____

_____

_____

_____

_____

_____

_____

_____

_____

_____

_____

_____

Practice until you are no longer afraid of your symptoms. During your practice do not try to reduce the anxiety in any way, either through any thinking methods, breathing activities, or any other relaxation behaviors. Trust that if you have done the work on the social anxiety mind game prior to this exercise, your anxiety will ebb on its own without help from you. Just keep practicing.

Face Your Fear of Positive Attention

Write down a list of situations that elicit positive attention that you are currently avoiding or enduring with a lot of discomfort.

1. _____
2. _____
3. _____
4. _____
5. _____
6. _____
7. _____

Next, write down some situations that will allow you to face your fear:

1. _____
2. _____
3. _____
4. _____
5. _____
6. _____
7. _____

Below are some examples of how to face your fear of positive attention:

- Dress up in attractive, stylish clothing or wear red lipstick.

- Talk about a success you have had personally or professionally.

- Talk about something that is going well in your life.

- Discuss a vacation you have taken, including showing off your vacation photos.

- If you have children, talk about their successes.

- If you have pets, talk about their positive qualities.

- Discuss something that you are looking forward to.

- Talk about a positive event you attended, such as a wedding, concert, play, etc.

You will often find that getting started is the hardest part. I encourage you to get going with whatever item scares you the least. Once you get going, there is often a sense of momentum that you build up and the rest of the items on your list are easier to approach. It is okay if this list makes you a little anxious – it should! Otherwise, it would not be worth your time to do it. Confronting anxiety involves raising your anxiety a little, so this just means you are doing it right!

How Improvisational Comedy Helps Quiet Social Anxiety

Improvisational comedy or "Improv" is a style of comedy that is unscripted and usually develops onstage from an audience suggestion. As such, it is unrehearsed, and creating it is frightening to almost everyone who is unfamiliar with this art form. Improv comedy is helpful for Social anxiety in the following ways:

1. It gives you permission to make mistakes. Yes, improv comedy celebrates mistakes, often with a loud cheer. This runs counter to social anxiety's notion that making a mistake is irreparable and intolerable. Once you play with improv comedy, you begin to notice that most mistakes are tolerable, that some go unnoticed, and that some turn into wonderful surprises. We once misheard a comedic suggestion from the audience, and what followed was an absurd scene that was simply fun to perform and that the audience loved.

2. Improv lets you be vulnerable and tolerate that

vulnerability. Improv is a real time team sport.
You do not know how it is going to go, and you
have to be there and risk looking foolish – which
makes everyone vulnerable to criticism. This addresses the fear of judgment, which is one of the
key fears of social anxiety.

3. Improv addresses our fears of not being likeable
    or valuable. A key aspect of improv comedy is
    supporting your partner or partners. As such,
    each scene is an opportunity to be seen, valued,
    and supported for your contribution.

CHAPTER XII.

Depression and Anxiety

"In the storm, our only anchor is hope." Laila Gifty Akita,
Pearls of Great Wisdom: Great Mind

Fighting your anxiety can feel exhausting, and it is common for someone who struggles with anxiety to also experience depression. It is estimated that as high a proportion as 60% of people who experience anxiety also experience depression (*Psychiatric Times, December 01, 2007 | Anxiety, Depression, Comorbidity In Psychiatry, Mood Disorders, Generalized Anxiety, Major Depressive Disorder, Dysthymia, by Oliver G. Cameron MD PhD, accessed September 28, 2016*).

Depression is defined by sad mood, difficulty enjoying activities that you typically find pleasurable, having a negative outlook about yourself and your future, sleep disturbance, weight gain or loss, and feelings of hopelessness, and for some people, it includes experiencing suicidal thoughts.

If you are struggling with depression, please know that you are not alone. If you experience suicidal thoughts or thoughts having to do with ending your life, please tell someone and seek professional help. You can gain support 24 hours / 7 days a week by calling a national suicide hotline. Below are the numbers for national suicide hotlines in the United States and Canada.

US number:
1-(800) SUICIDE or 1-(800) 784-2433

Canada:
National Suicide Prevention Lifeline:
1-(800) 273-TALK

If you experience depression symptoms without suicidal thoughts, there are a number of strategies you can use to help yourself:

1. Exercise. Try to get at least 30 minutes of moderate physical activity per day. If possible, have it take place outdoors.

2. Create a list of pleasurable activities and schedule

at least one per day. Look forward to this and savor it. Some examples are:

- Drink a cup of your favorite herbal tea

- Get a manicure or do an at-home manicure

- Take a long bubble bath

- Read for pleasure

- Get a massage

- Schedule time to spend with a friend

- Buy fresh or potted flowers

- Have some creative time: paint, take photographs, or make a collage

- Sit in a café and people watch

- Go to your favorite museum

- Cook your favorite meal

- Play with your pet

- Look at photos of your last vacation

- Play an instrument

- Listen to your favorite music

- Plan your next vacation

- Play with your children

- Plant a garden

- Enjoy looking at the stars at night

- Watch the beauty of a sunrise or sunset

You may wish to enhance this list by adding your own favorite activities.

3. Get some social support.
   Spend some time with the people you enjoy most. Chat about how you feel and what you need. Chat about what you want and hope for. Enjoy being and connecting with someone you love.

4. Volunteer.
   Volunteering has been shown to have a positive effect on our mood. Sometimes devoting a bit of time to helping someone else can change our outlook and give us perspective. Look for volunteer organizations in your area. Hospitals, civic organizations, and religious institutions are a good place to start exploring your options.

5. Stay Active.
   Depression lies to you by encouraging you to hibernate, stay at home, nap, sleep excessively, and avoid people and activities you used to enjoy. Do not fall for it – it is likely to make you feel

worse. Get out of bed, go see your friends, and stay engaged even when you do not particularly feel like it. You are likely to feel better when you stay engaged rather than when you are isolated or withdrawn.

6. Keep a Gratitude Journal.

   Write down everything that you are grateful for, no matter how small. For example:

   - My health

   - My supportive family

   - My child

   - That I learned how to ski

   - That I am employed

   - That I don't have to worry about access to food, shelter, and clean water

   - That I can make a great baked eggplant

   - That I am married to a person I love

   - That I had the best chocolate soufflé cake last night

   - That my body is able to move so that I can run and play sports

- That I live in a country where everyone has a right to an education

- That I get to see how beautiful fall is in the Midwest

- That I got to take an unexpectedly long lunch

- That I got to return a few phone calls while waiting in line

- That I am able to enjoy summer peaches and plums

- That a stranger gave me a friendly smile this morning

- That I know how to swim and I enjoy it

- My pet

- My ability to make a great collage

- That my sneakers get me through some tough runs

Keep adding to your personal list daily until you reach at least 50. Then, look over your list every two to three days and add at least one item each time.

Helping Depression Through Awakening Your Sense of Awe

The feeling of awe is that combination of amazement and wonder that children enjoy and experience every day. As adults those experiences become more infrequent. The good news is that we can awaken a sense of awe through very simple experiences. If you struggle with depression, experiencing a sense of awe can help you in the following ways:

1. You experience and connect with something larger than yourself and your struggles. For example, being in nature can often lead to experiencing a sense of awe through noticing the many ways nature is expansive and surprising. The next time you are walking or hiking, notice what strikes you; the vast skies, a beautiful waterway, a mountain landscape, trees and their colorful foliage.

2. You fly in the face of gray; depression has one offering on the menu – bleak, gray days ahead. Give it something of contrast – if you live in a big city with sparse access to nature, look at

landscape photography, visit animals in the zoo, a botanical garden, or a butterfly sanctuary. If you are fortunate to live in an area with plenty of parks and easy access to natural vistas, take a walk and notice all the colors that nature offers, all the ways it stretches. **TIP: Take a camera with you and capture what you see.**

3. You begin to tap into a sense of joy. Awe is a positive emotion, and feeling it can jumpstart and kindle a different energy. I encourage you to play a game of trying to find awe in as many places as possible over the next week. Feel free to include places and situations beyond the natural world; enjoy a magnificent cityscape, watch a professional athlete compete, marvel at someone's personality trait that you admire. Notice how you feel.

CHAPTER XIII

The Role of Medication

"Laughter is the best medicine - unless you're diabetic, then insulin comes pretty high on the list." —*Jasper Carrott*

Medication may or may not have a role in your treatment. If your symptoms are very severe, if they interfere with a major area of your life that is critical (you are unable to work, for example), or if you feel that you are in crisis, it makes sense for you to get an evaluation for psychotropic medication. Medication can serve as an adjunct to you working on your anxiety. However, medication is not a stand-alone solution, as it does not resolve the issue; it just helps with current symptoms for as long as you take the medication.

There are different classes of medication: long acting and short acting. Long acting medications take time to work and are taken daily regardless of the symptoms you experience. Short-acting medications are taken intermittently at symptom onset, although they are sometimes prescribed to take every day.

Long-acting medications that are prescribed for anxiety management are typically in the category of Selective Serotonin Reuptake Inhibitors or SSRIs. SSRIs work by making the neurotransmitter serotonin more available in the brain by delaying its reuptake. Commonly prescribed SSRIs include fluoxetine (Prozac), sertraline (Zoloft), fluvoxamine (Luvox), paroxetine (Paxil), escitalopram (Lexapro), and citalopram (Celexa). SSRIs work by inhibiting the reuptake of serotonin at the nerve synapse, which makes the serotonin available to your nervous system for a longer period of time than it otherwise would be. This, in turn, has a positive effect on lowering your anxiety. SSRIs similarly have a positive effect on depressive symptoms. If you are someone who experiences anxiety and depression, this class of medication can treat both symptoms. Typically, this class of medication affects your overall anxiety level and makes it easier for you to tolerate situations that were previously very anxiety-provoking. The medication is non-addictive and will not take away all of your anxiety. This means that you are able to take this class of medication while gradually facing your fears. The medication alone is unlikely to be the entire treatment plan, as typically the effect of the medication wears off when you discontinue taking it. This means that if you did not engage in any other work to manage your anxiety, your symptoms are likely to return once you discontinue the medication. On the other hand, if you have engaged in some work on the anxiety mind game and have been able to face your fears, then you are in a good position to continue with your gains even after you discontinue your medication. SSRIs can often be another tool in treating your anxiety.

Short-acting medications usually prescribed for anxiety fall into two classes: benzodiazepines and beta blockers. Commonly prescribed benzodiazepines are Alprazolam (Xanax), Lorazepam (Ativan), Clonazepam (Klonopin), and Diazepam (Valium). Benzodiazepines work to calm the central nervous system by enhancing the work of a calming neurotransmitter called Gamma Amino Butyric Acid or GABA. Benzodiazepines have a risk of building tolerance, and there is a risk for physical addiction, particularly when used long term.

Beta blockers such as Inderal are beta-adrenergic antagonists. They block the effects of norepinephrine and adrenaline, a stress hormone, and are therefore some-times prescribed for panic attacks, because they reduce the physical symptoms associated with the fight or flight response, such as rapid heartbeat. Beta blockers are not physically addictive, however, there is potential for psy-chological addiction; we can feel that we are not able to function adequately without them.

Unless you are in crisis, short-acting medication is not your best bet. In particular, if you struggle with panic or phobias, it can actually work against you. This happens because they prevent you from fully experiencing your anxiety on demand. While that may seem like a wonderful idea, in reality it functions much like avoidance. That is, it blocks you from experiencing your body's own anxiety reduction mechanism in action. Only a licensed medical professional can prescribe and dispense medication, but I encourage you to discuss your concerns regarding short-acting medication with your doctor if that is the recommendation that you receive. If you are thinking of making any changes to your existing medication regimen, please discuss it with your medical professional. Trying to make medication changes without the guidance of a medical professional may result in you experiencing adverse reactions.

Many people do not want to take medication or have it be part of the treatment picture. If you are not in a serious emotional crisis, it is entirely possible that you will beat anxiety without medication. If you are already prescribed benzodiazepines or beta blockers for anxiety and are concerned about their effects or feel you may have developed dependence on or addiction to them, please consult your healthcare provider. If you are not sure which option is best for you, a consultation with a qualified mental health professional can often provide much-needed clarity.

CHAPTER XIV

Troubleshooting: How to Get Through Your Stuck Spots

"If you're trying to achieve, there will be roadblocks. I've had them; everybody has had them. But obstacles don't have to stop you. If you run into a wall, don't turn around and give up. Figure out how to climb it, go through it, or work around it." —Michael Jordan

Are you expecting changes to happen quickly?

As with any new skill you learn, you will notice that some skills are gained faster than others. When we make rapid gains, we typically feel positive and satisfied. When positive changes come more slowly, we tend to feel deflated and may even think of giving up. This points to a problem with regard to our expectations. Most people start working on their anxiety years after the initial problem developed. How could something that has taken years to evolve be changed very quickly? It probably cannot, and it is to be expected that as you are developing new skills you will have to practice self compassion when those desired skills take longer to develop. This is the time for kindness and patience toward yourself. You are not necessarily supposed to master all of these skills quickly. Rather, you are embarking on a journey of mastery and building new life-long habits, and that can take some time.

Are you expecting that you will master every skill easily?

Some of the skills that you are learning are just going to be easier for you to develop and hone than others. For example, for some of my clients, relaxation is a very easy skill to acquire. However, for others, it is an uphill battle! If you are used to anxiety running your mind with the pace of a high-speed jet, then the very act of relaxation can feel extremely uncomfortable, if not outright terrifying. During those moments it is important that you do not treat your difficulty in developing a particular skill as a lack of progress. Rather, I would like for you to approach it as a brand new language, one that you are completely unfamiliar with and one that will take a bit of time and practice to learn and use easily and comfortably.

Is judgment getting in your way?

During times of struggle, judgment tends to appear with a vengeance. It is important that you are mindful of the noise that this creates in your mind and that you do not start criticizing or blaming yourself. Treat the noise as you treat street noise in a busy city; it is supposed to be there, but you get to decide how much you pay attention to the noise – whether you want to focus on that noise of judgment or on something you find more valuable. When your attention wanders, which it may, just return it back to what you were doing beforehand.

Are you staying open to the possibility of change?

When I first suggest to my clients that their life may feel very different in a matter of months, it is often hard for them to imagine. After all, anxiety and its habitual blueprint have become all too familiar, and any deviation is met with skepticism. I invite you to stay open to the possibility that you may not always feel this way. This is particularly challenging when we encounter a roadblock on our journey to overcome anxiety and panic. Please remember that envisioning your goal will serve you in staying the course. You will truly believe it only after the change has already happened. Until then, I encourage you to take it on faith that with practice, anxiety and panic can be overcome!

Facing your fears: are your exposures too difficult?

Oftentimes if you have done the work on your thoughts and beliefs and have difficulty facing your fears, it is because your practice opportunities are too challenging. The solution is to break them down into even easier and more manageable situations. For example, if it is difficult for you to start practicing flirting with people who you find attractive, you may wish to start with making eye contact first. Then you could move into making eye contact and smiling. Next time you may try to make eye contact, smile and say "Hello." At your next practice opportunity, you may decide to move on to paying someone a compliment.

Only after all of those steps have been completed will you move on to flirting.

Are you creating enough momentum?

It is possible to create your list of practice opportunities or exposures that are just right for you and yet still experience difficulties getting started or progressing through your list. If you determined that the exposures are not too difficult, momentum could be the problem. When we practice exposures, if we do just one exposure and wait a few days, it is often difficult to sustain the energy and motivation from the prior success we had. Success here is defined as completing the exposure or practice opportunity. For this reason, I will recommend that you create practice opportunities that allow you to "stack" your exposures so that you complete three in a row. This method allows you to generate the momentum you need to continue and will eliminate the temptation to write off any single successful exposure as a fluke. What you are creating when you are stacking exposures are the conditions that allow you to get started without feeling like you have to ramp up to doing the exposure each time. Stacking exposures this way and performing them for several consecutive days is even more powerful and will help you progress faster.

7 Ways to Become More Resilient in the Face of Setbacks

1. Adopt a hopeful outlook. Optimism has been linked to resilience. If this does not come naturally to you, ask yourself how a more optimistic friend would look at the situation.

2. Build good supportive relationships. It has been found that people who have good relationships with family and friends are happier and more resilient.

3. Remove the crisis from setbacks. Getting through a difficult situation is tough enough without feeling the pressure and urgency of overreaction. Try to focus on action instead.

4. Take excellent care of yourself. When you get adequate rest, nutrition, and exercise, setbacks become easier to weather.

5. Look at setbacks as a chance to grow and learn something about yourself. People who adopt this attitude are able to see the situation with a broader perspective.

6. Develop and support a positive view of yourself. Remind yourself that you have strengths and re- sources that will help you get through tough situ- ations and setbacks. Make a list of your strengths and refer to it periodically.

7. Work on goals and take action. Having personal goals and taking steps to remedy or better your situation has been linked with resilience building.

PART 4

LIFELONG ANXIETY MANAGEMENT PLAN IN ACTION

"Everything in the universe has a purpose. Indeed, the invisible intelligence that flows through everything in a purposeful fashion is also flowing through you." —Wayne Dyer

CHAPTER XV.

Maintain Your
Gains for Life

Now that you have gone over the steps needed and developed an action plan to overcome panic and social anxiety, we will focus the final part of the book on lifelong anxiety management. You will learn how to maintain the gains that you have made. You will also learn how to develop lifelong habits that help maintain and continue to grow your progress in managing panic and social anxiety.

Self-care

Good self-care is essential to lifelong anxiety management. This means total self-care. Self care involves dedicating time and resources to meet the following personal needs: sleep, rest, exercise, nutrition, connection, and spirituality. Self-care is not the same as being selfish. In fact, it is the opposite. When you consistently practice good self-care, you become more available to other people and your most important relationships.

Sleep

Take a look at how much sleep you are getting. Most adults need seven to nine hours per night. If you are not getting enough sleep, your hormonal levels, your mood, and your anxiety levels can be affected. How much sleep is enough for you? That depends. Try to let yourself wake up without an alarm for a few days. What do you notice? Do you feel sleepy after you have gotten up and had breakfast? If so, and if you are getting less than the recommended amount of sleep, try adding thirty minutes each night for a few nights and seeing how you feel. If you are still tired, you may want to consult with your physician, who may recommend checking into your sleep quality and perhaps doing a sleep study to rule out a sleep disorder.

If you have difficulty falling asleep at night or going back to sleep after waking up in the middle of the night, try the following exercise.

Getting to Sleep Exercise

Get into your preferred comfortable sleeping position so that you do not have to shift or move while doing this exercise. Close your eyes. Starting at the top of your head, go through this sequence of <u>slowly</u> repeating the following to yourself, repeating the sequence several times if needed:

- My forehead is tired, heavy, and sleepy and cannot move.

- My eyes are tired, heavy, and sleepy and cannot move.

- My cheeks are tired, heavy, and sleepy and cannot move.

- My chin is tired, heavy, and sleepy and cannot move.

- My head is tired, heavy, and sleepy and cannot move.

- My neck is tired, heavy, and sleepy and cannot move.

- My shoulders are tired, heavy, and sleepy and cannot move.

- My upper arms are tired, heavy, and sleepy and cannot move.

- My lower arms are tired, heavy, and sleepy and cannot move.

- My hands are tired, heavy, and sleepy and cannot move.

- My chest is tired, heavy, and sleepy and cannot move.

- My back is tired, heavy, and sleepy and cannot move.

- My stomach is tired, heavy and sleepy and cannot move.

- My hips are tired, heavy, and sleepy and cannot move.

- My upper legs are tired, heavy, and sleepy and cannot move.

- My lower legs are tired, heavy, and sleepy and cannot move.

- My ankles are tired, heavy, and sleepy and cannot move.

- My feet are tired, heavy, and sleepy and cannot move.

- My entire body is tired, heavy, and sleepy and cannot move.

Practice this technique for several nights to become comfortable with it.

Another factor to look at if you are having difficulty with sleep is your sleep routine, or what psychologists call "sleep hygiene." Several factors contribute to good sleep hygiene.

1. Keep your bedroom activity restricted to sleep, sex, and relaxation. This means keeping work or any other activities restricted to outside the bedroom. If you live in a studio apartment, you may wish to consider restricting other activity to outside the actual bed.

2. Have a winding down routine that is similar day to day. This means that about one hour before bed, you engage in winding down and low-key or relaxing activities. For example, this may include reading, meditation, or taking a bath.

3. If you have difficulty with sleep, it may be important to power off your electronic devices, such as smartphones, laptops, and tablets, one hour prior to bedtime.

4. Consider your eating and drinking habits and limit alcohol before bed. Eating a heavy meal before bedtime can also interfere with your sleep. Try having an earlier dinner and consuming less food closer to bedtime. Limit caffeine to the early part of the day, particularly if you are sensitive to it.

5. Limit napping, and keep your naps to ninety minutes or less if you find that they are necessary or enjoyable.

6. Wake up at a consistent time every day, even on weekends.

Diet

Proper nutrition is important. Make sure you are getting the right balance of proteins, carbohydrates, and fats. Try to cut down on processed foods and eat plenty of fresh fruits and vegetables. Eat regular meals so you do not get hypoglycemia (low blood sugar). Low blood sugar can mimic symptoms of anxiety and panic, such as lightheadedness, nausea, and dizziness – therefore it often escalates into anxiety or panic symptoms for individuals who are prone to anxiety. This can be easily prevented with regular, balanced meals.

Exercise

Exercise is known to boost mood and decrease stress. Certain types of exercise also have mind-body benefits. Yoga, tai chi, and Pilates, as well as other forms of exercise that emphasize the mind-body connection, are great to include in your regimen. I am a particular fan of yoga, which teaches you breathing, meditation, and mindfulness. Try out a few classes and see what works for you.

A Full Life

The truth is the definition of a "full" life widely varies. What I will tell you is that anxiety tends to rear its ugly head when we are ignoring something important in our life. In order to get a well-rounded assessment of how you are doing, please consider your answers when completing the following "My Life Values Exercise."

My Life Values Exercise

Please consider how well you would rate your satisfaction in the following areas:

Work   1 2 3 4 5 6 7 8 9 10

Family Relationships   1 2 3 4 5 6 7 8 9 10

Romantic Relationship   1 2 3 4 5 6 7 8 9 10

Friendships   1 2 3 4 5 6 7 8 9 10

Hobbies   1 2 3 4 5 6 7 8 9 10

Exercise   1 2 3 4 5 6 7 8 9 10

Physical Health   1 2 3 4 5 6 7 8 9 10

Emotional Health   1 2 3 4 5 6 7 8 9 10

Socializing   1 2 3 4 5 6 7 8 9 10

Spirituality   1 2 3 4 5 6 7 8 9 10

Activities that give you a sense of meaning	1 2 3 4 5 6 7 8 9 10
Activities that give you a sense of connection	1 2 3 4 5 6 7 8 9 10
Activities that are relaxing, recharging, or rejuvenating	1 2 3 4 5 6 7 8 9 10

Please reflect on your ratings. Is there an area, or several, that you rated lower than you would like? How can you make room for it in your already busy schedule? Can you schedule a specific time in your calendar to act on it? It is unlikely that you will master anxiety management if you are ignoring an important area in your life. We all have to decide what makes a meaningful and full life. Asking those questions, while challenging, is also the very thing that leads us to discover the answers and contributes to lower anxiety in the long run.

Anxiety as a Fellow Traveler

There are some experts out there who suggest learning to love your anxiety.

I think that is a tall order. To this day I have not met a single person, personally or professionally, myself included, who has had a desire to do this. I do not think this is necessary. All that is required is that you accept that when anxiety shows up, you can say to this uninvited guest, "You are here, and I will follow what I intend to do regardless of your presence here, so come along if you wish – it will not deter me!" It is about accepting your anxiety as a fellow traveler through life – one that at times is needed to guide you to the right path and at other times is merely alongside you.

There is a difference between taking your anxiety along while pursuing the activities that you intend and distracting yourself with activity. If you have ever tried to distract yourself from your anxiety, you know that it does not work. At the very least, it does not work for long. And yet, we often hear this well-meaning advice, "Just distract yourself! Stay busy!"

Being busy is always good – isn't it? Not really. Trying to stay active in order to distract yourself from your anxiety means that anxiety is in charge. You read and you wonder, "Is it over? When will it go away?" You go for a run and you ask yourself, "Am I still anxious or is it over?" Anxiety is calling the shots – it is the compass and the guide. Referencing your anxiety by asking these questions is akin to asking its permission. This means that you have now stepped down from being in charge and will ask anxiety when it is okay for you to proceed, relax, etc. I want you to take charge; I want you to empower yourself with the idea that anxiety will only be in charge if you decide so. Engage in whatever activity you think is valuable, not to distract, but to attain what you consider to be a valued path or direction.

Unhelpful Habits

There are unhelpful habits that can trigger or perpetuate anxiety.

1. **Caffeine**

    Caffeine is a stimulant. In high doses it is neurotoxic. Some people are sensitive to caffeine and may show a reaction to a very small dose, for example a few pieces of chocolate. Some foods and beverages that contain caffeine are: coffee, tea, colas, energy drinks, and chocolate. What caffeine does is stimulate the production of cortisol, a stress hormone. Since your response to caffeine is unique, please notice your reaction to it and respond accordingly. If you are having repeated panic attacks, it is a good idea to cut down. If you have been ingesting caffeine daily and wish to cut down, please do not do it cold turkey. Stopping caffeine use abruptly can lead to rebound anxiety, so a gradual approach is always recommended.

2. **Nicotine**

    Nicotine is a stimulant, and although people may use it to relax, it actually increases your anxiety by stimulating cortisol production. Similarly to caffeine, cutting down gradually is advised in order to prevent rebound anxiety.

3. Alcohol

Alcohol is a depressant. Although many people use alcohol to relax and even reduce their anxiety, alcohol also raises cortisol levels. This is particularly apparent after overindulging in alcohol or during the "hangover" period. Every single person who I have seen in my consultation room has noticed this effect. How sensitive you are to alcohol varies, so please notice your own response – some people can have a reaction after only one or two drinks.

4. Other drugs

Other illicit as well as prescription drugs and supplements can trigger anxiety. This includes certain vitamins in high doses, such as Vitamin B-12 and other "natural" supplements. Please consult your doctor or pharmacist if you are concerned about a drug or supplement that you are taking.

5. Perfectionism

You may be surprised to see perfectionism included on the list of unhelpful habits. The truth is perfectionism really does get us off track in terms of anxiety management. We tend to set unrealistic expectations when we use perfectionism as the standard. We tend to feel bad about what we accomplished. And we tend to miss the point of engaging in an imperfect process as an imperfect human being and all the learning that comes along with it. I encourage you to give up perfectionism as quickly as possible. You will get better in terms of managing anxiety and you may have fantastic results, however it will never be perfect – nor does it have to be! An alternative view is just to focus on doing your imperfect best in any situation.

6. **Procrastination**

Putting off tasks, assignments, and life goals can make us anxious. Procrastination is the simplest and most common form of avoidance. Therefore, like all avoidance, it will raise our anxiety, and when practiced repeatedly, it will cement the anxiety cycle. It usually shows up in three areas: to-dos, difficult conversations, and life goals.

Your To Do List

Take a look at your to do list. Are there certain things that you need to deal with? Do you need to make that doctor's appointment that you have been putting off because you are scared you may get bad news? Do you need to take your car in for a safety check? Do you need to mail some letters or write an important e-mail?

Write down everything you need to do, prioritize in order of urgency and importance, and then start tackling them one by one by putting each on your calendar like an appointment with yourself.

1. _____
   Date & Time _____

2. _____
   Date & Time _____

3. _____
   Date & Time _____

4. _____
   Date & Time _____

5. _____
   Date & Time _____

6. _____
   Date & Time _____

7. _____
   Date & Time _____

Difficult Conversations

Write down any difficult conversations that you need to have. Do you need to fire your dog-walker? Call the phone company to get a better rate? Ask your mate to pitch in more around the house? Ask your boss for a raise? Start with the one that is the most pressing, or that you find the easiest to do, and work down your list.

The Conversations I Need to Have Are:

1. _____
   Date & Time _____
2. _____
   Date & Time _____
3. _____
   Date & Time _____
4. _____
   Date & Time _____
5. _____
   Date & Time _____
6. _____
   Date & Time _____
7. _____
   Date & Time _____

Life Goals

Write down your life goals and dreams. Take a look at the list and see if there is something that you have not attended to. There may be several items that feel important. Use your gut to determine what you think you need to act on first. Did you always want to travel abroad? Are you looking to live in a different city? Have you been dreaming about completing your college degree or going to graduate school? Is there a certain hobby that you have wanted to try if you could muster the courage: dancing, learning a language, surfing?

While this may take a bit of self-reflection on your part, it is well worth it! You deserve a life that is well aligned with your values and interests. If anxiety has been keeping you hostage, it is time to fight back. Take a step into the direction of valued living. Accept the imperfection of trial and error and the possibility that you may not love everything you try. Add a bit of playfulness to this experiment and you will find that it can be fun to explore!

The Life Goals I Would Like to Act on Are:

1. _____

   Date & Time _____

2. _____

   Date & Time _____

3. _____

   Date & Time _____

4. _____

   Date & Time _____

5. _____

   Date & Time _____

6. _____

Date & Time _____

7. _____

Date & Time _____

8. Rushing

Rushing is inevitably likely to make us anxious. Look at when this happens in your life, and try to plan a few extra minutes so that rushing is an exception and not a way of life for you. In our busy lives this may seem impossible, but I promise that if you look at your day, you can probably find pockets of activity that can be removed to create this extra time.

9. Impatience

I get it. You have been struggling for a while and you just want this anxiety and panic to stop and you want it to stop now! You have spent a long time, your patience is long gone, and you sometimes feel like you cannot take another moment of this. The time is now and there is no time to wait. This sense of urgency is undeniable, understandable, and it is also how panic and anxiety get to win.

You are not looking for immediate relief here – that is what you get with avoidance – and we know that has not helped you one bit! We are looking at the long game here: your life. It is worth it to take the time you need to beat panic and anxiety, and for that you will have to be patient. For that, my dear reader, you will have to put the immediate urgency aside and really take in, learn, and practice your skills. To really get better, you will have to invest your time, energy, and patience in yourself. Even when you feel tired, impatient, and want it to stop, I will ask you to take a few breaths and practice the next step in this next moment. Really be here in practicing and receiving this information and mastering the skills. Observe your impatience without judgment when it shows up, and go alongside it to do what you need to do. You can do this!

Welcome Pause Exercise

This exercise is intended to help with impatience in situations where your day is interrupted and you may be forced to wait or stop what you are doing. A few examples are: waiting in a long line, being stuck on a train, bus, or in heavy traffic, or waiting at the airport when your flight is delayed. These conditions are likely to trigger impatience even in the most well-tempered individuals. I encourage you to begin treating these situations as opportunities for practicing impatience tolerance.

The next time you find yourself in one of these situations and are feeling the pangs of impatience, I encourage you to say to yourself, "this is a welcome pause in my busy life," and to begin to treat it as such. In those moments I would like you to take a few slow abdominal breaths and enjoy this pause. Next, treat this as an opportunity to enjoy this moment as you wish; listen to music, read, doodle, or just take a relaxing break. Trust that there is a place for this interruption or delay in your day, and make the best of it by slowing down a bit rather than running ragged in the direction impatience is sure to drag you – if you let it. After each practice, observe how you feel.

Helpful Habits

Relaxation Practice
A regular relaxation practice is essential to lifelong anxiety management. There are many ways to achieve this. The simplest one is to practice diaphragmatic breathing for ten minutes a day. Other ways to include relaxation in your life include Progressive Muscle Relaxation, visualization, meditation, and the use of affirmations.

Diaphragmatic Breathing
Diaphragmatic breathing is also known as abdominal

or "belly" breathing. To practice this, lie down on your back with your hands clasped over your stomach. Take a breath in and watch what happens. If you are doing this properly, the stomach goes up on an inhale and goes down on an exhale. If you are doing the reverse, practice until it becomes comfortable, keeping your hands over your abdominals. Practice for ten minutes each day.

Progressive Muscle Relaxation

Progressive Muscle Relaxation is an easy-to-learn technique that can be very relaxing and can be used before you go to bed to help you fall asleep, or at any time that you feel tense or stressed. You will sequentially tense and relax a few selected muscle groups and take a diaphragmatic breath in between each one. Make sure that you tighten the muscle to the point of tension, but not strain. Your goal is two-fold: you will be relaxing your body, and you will also build awareness of your body's tension and relaxation states over time. This will help you notice when you are feeling tense so you can activate your relaxation response.

To begin, sit comfortably in a chair with your arms and legs uncrossed, and close your eyes. Start from your tiptoes and move upwards in your body.

Progressive Muscle Relaxation Sequence

1. Tense and relax your toes by scrunching them.

Let it go.
Take a breath in and take a breath out.

2. Lift up on your heels to tense your calves. Let it go.
   Take a breath in and take a breath out.

3. Press both feet firmly into the floor to tense the quadriceps. Let it go.
   Take a breath in and take a breath out.

4. Tense your buttocks. Let it go.
   Take a breath in and take a breath out.

5. Suck your stomach in. Let it go.
   Take a breath in and take a breath out.

6. Stick your chest out. Let it go.
   Take a breath in and take a breath out.

7. Raise your shoulders to your ears. Let it go.
   Take a breath in and take a breath out.

8. Clench your fists to tense your forearms. Let it go.
   Take a breath in and take a breath out.

9. Lift up an imaginary barbell to tense the biceps. Let it go.

Take a breath in and take a breath out.

10. Scrunch your face towards your nose. Let it go.
    Take a breath in and take a breath out.

11. Raise your eyebrows. Let it go.
    Take a breath in and take a breath out.

12. Check in with your jaw (that you are not clenching). If you are clenching, part your lips slightly and touch the roof of your mouth with the tip of your tongue at the point where the gum-line meets the inside of your upper front teeth.
    Take a breath in and take a breath out.

13. Check in with your eyelids (that you are not pulling them shut).
    Take a breath in and take a breath out.

    Keep breathing for a few minutes after you have finished. If you would like, do a second round followed by a few minutes of diaphragmatic breathing. Practice nightly for three weeks and then as needed.

Visualization

Visualization is a powerful tool to aid in stress management and is a great addition to your relaxation practice. I will teach you two techniques. Try them both and pick one that you will practice for a few weeks. Then, try the next one for a few weeks.

The first exercise is called the three-minute vacation. This is a great exercise to practice anytime you need a break, but do not have the luxury of time. It only takes a few minutes, and when practiced regularly, it can really reduce your stress level. Find a quiet space where you can relax and will not be interrupted. Next, set a timer for three minutes.

Three-Minute Vacation Exercise

Close your eyes and picture a place you find relaxing. This could be a real place you have visited or a purely imagined place. Try to pick a place that does not have any unpleasant associations with it. Now picture what it looks like. If it is a beach, describe the color of the water, the sand, any wildlife and plant life you see. Look at the sky and all of the shapes of the clouds. After you have finished, tune in to any sounds you hear. Are the birds chirping? Can you hear the waves crashing? Can you hear the sound of children laughing in the distance? Now focus on your physical sensations. Can you feel the sun warming your skin? Can you feel the breeze gently tousling your hair? Are your toes touching the grainy sand? Next, tune into the scents around you. Can you smell the ocean? Are there any flowers blooming nearby? Is there a smell of barbequed food carried by the breeze? Can you taste anything? Are you sipping lemonade or snacking on something? Hold this picture in your mind as you feel relaxed and breathe diaphragmatically for a few minutes. Check in with how you feel, slowly open your eyes, and remember that you can carry this relaxed feeling with you into the rest of your day.

Another technique you can practice is called the paint yourself relaxed exercise.

Paint Yourself Relaxed Exercise

Sit in a comfortable position with your arms and legs uncrossed. Close your eyes. Picture a warm-toned paint color, like yellow, orange, or coral. Start at the tips of your toes and imagine the color slowly painting and spreading upwards, with each move spreading a warm relaxing sensation over your body. Starting at the toes, picture it moving upwards over your ankles, calves, knees, thighs, hips, abdomen, the chest, and your shoulders. Picture it spreading relaxing warmth down both arms: your upper arms, lower arms, wrists, hands, and down towards the very tips of your fingertips. Now picture it going back up and moving across your neck and your face, all the way up towards the top of your scalp. You are now wrapped in warmth. The warmth is at just the right temperature for you. Stay here with your eyes closed and practice diaphragmatic breathing for a few minutes. Slowly open your eyes after you have finished. Then check in with how you feel. Use this anytime you feel stressed or need a break. This is also a good technique to use before bed to help you fall asleep.

Meditation

There has been a lot of research on how good meditation is for both your physical and mental health. The biggest stumbling block I see to starting a meditation practice seems to be expectations. It is often recommended that you start meditating in ten-minute increments. Ten minutes of meditation is a long time if you have never practiced it. I invite you to start with a goal of one minute. There are many resources out there if you wish to delve deeper into meditation. You can go to a Buddhist temple, a yoga studio, or a freestanding meditation center to take a class.

I will start you off with a one-minute meditation primer here, and let you decide how to pursue your meditation study and practice further.

Sit down in a comfortable seated position. If you do not practice yoga regularly, I would advise you to do what is called western style meditation. Rather than sitting on a cushion on the floor, you can sit in a comfortable chair, preferably one with armrests. Start by sitting with arms and legs uncrossed and your eyes closed. Set a timer for 60 seconds. After one minute becomes easy for you to complete, you can add a minute and work up to two minutes, three minutes, and so on.

With your eyes closed, I would like you to take a detached stance towards your thoughts. It is unrealistic to expect yourself to be completely free of thought and so a detached stance allows you to experience thoughts and images without getting involved or embroiled in their meaning or consequence. I would like you to think of your thoughts like clouds passing over a blue sky. When we glance upwards, we may have a thought about a particular shape of the cloud, but it rarely sticks with us and we usually are able to watch the clouds go by. Breathe as you do this, using the diaphragmatic breathing technique. Notice any effects after you have finished. A meditation practice takes a long time to feel like second nature, so it is important to be gentle with yourself as you are learning it and to practice self-compassion when it does not come easily.

With repeated practice, you may notice that not only does it get easier to do, but that you are also able to feel the full relaxation effects of it at a deeper level. Although this is the most advanced of all relaxation techniques, and can take a bit of effort to learn, it can also be the most powerful. Because you are starting off slowly and practicing for only a minute at a time, it is advised if you can, you try to practice it two to three times a day to aid in learning this skill.

Affirmations

Affirmations are positive statements that you repeat to yourself with the purpose of motivating you and encouraging your progress. Affirmations are not simply changing an unwelcome reality by replacing it with a positive one. The latter type of replacement affirmation is a white lie. You are too smart to believe it, and so it simply cannot and does not work! For example, telling yourself: "I am a relaxed person with little anxiety" while in the midst of dealing with strong symptoms of anxiety is a type of replacement affirmation I advise against. Most people who did not have a good experience with affirmations have tried using replacement affirmations.

Affirmations are in the present tense, future-oriented, and use active language. Passive language affirmations imply that a solution will occur with no input from you. As with most things in life, positive change is unlikely to happen by a stroke of luck. We have to take steps towards our goals, and so our affirmations need to use the active tense.

Example of a passive affirmation: "A peaceful life will soon be mine."

Example of an active affirmation: "Each day I am taking steps and learning to better manage my anxiety."

Take a moment to develop an active affirmation for yourself below:

_____

_____

_____

_____

_____

_____

_____

I suggest that you practice your affirmation daily, either first thing in the morning or once in the evening. Practice for several weeks before assessing the effects.

Assertiveness

Assertiveness is the ability to ask for what you need and to be able to say "no" in order to set appropriate limits and boundaries. Many people with anxiety have difficulty in one or more areas of assertiveness. Please reflect on how assertive you are able to be in your life by looking at a list of the following assertive actions:

I am able to say "no" when I need to.

I am able to turn down an invitation.

I am able to resist a high-pressure salesperson.

I am able to ask for a favor from a friend or family member.

I am able to take time off for self-care without feeling guilty.

I am able to address hurt feelings in my relationships.

I am able to request an apology when I need to.

I am able to speak up about my preferences and likes.

I feel like I can get my needs met in my important relationships.

If you answered, "yes" to all of the questions above—good for you!

If not, consider working on developing your assertiveness skills in those areas. Start by making a list of all the assertiveness tasks that you would like to work on. Next, prioritize them from lowest to highest in difficulty. Finally, start going through your list by tackling the easiest tasks first and moving on to the more challenging ones. Please keep in mind that you are building new habits here and be kind to yourself if you falter.

Assertiveness Skills I Need to Work on Are:

_____
_____
_____
_____
_____
_____
_____
_____
_____

Being Present

Being present simply means allowing your attention to remain in the moment, rather than focusing on future or past events. Anxiety usually steals your attention to focus on some future undesirable and frightening scenario. When we feel down or depressed, we may replay a past scenario in our minds. In both cases, we are losing precious moments in our life that we will never get back. The only way to change this is to tune back in, starting at the moment that we realize that we have been anywhere other than the present. If you are looking for help in developing this skill, meditation is a great way to hone it.

Humor

Humor can be your secret weapon against anxiety. It is impossible to find something genuinely funny and to be scared of it at the same time. Anxiety makes you feel like the world, your life, and virtually any decision you make are so serious! Things feel so heavy and important that we start losing perspective and missing out on the lighter side of things. Let's flip anxiety on its axis! The next time you feel this heavy feeling of dread, weightiness, or nervous anticipation, try to find something funny in it. Draw a caricature of it; imagine a cartoon voice describing your fear, or a sitcom written about your situation. Anything that can get you laughing is a good start!

Decrease Anxiety with Cartooning Exercise

Anxiety often feels heavy and sounds dire and serious in its warnings. This exercise is designed to bring some levity to it. Imagine that your anxiety is a cartoon character. Picture what it would look like and what it would sound like. Please draw or describe it in the space below. This drawing is for your eyes only, so feel free to experiment, and ignore any artistic self-judgment that may show up.

If my anxiety were a cartoon character it would look like (describe in words or draw a picture):

_____

_____

_____

_____

_____

_____

_____

_____

_____

_____

If my anxiety were a cartoon character it would sound like:

_____

_____

_____

_____

_____

_____

_____

Next, using the cartoon voice, say a few things that anxiety tells you out loud.

> For example: "Even though it is untrue that you can pass out from a panic attack, I still think it might happen," or "I cannot read other people's minds, but I am pretty sure they are judging me anyway! I should think of all the possible negative things they are thinking about me." Check in with how you feel after this exercise. When I do this exercise with my clients, they invariably start giggling. It is quite freeing to laugh at our own anxiety because we start taking its warning messages a lot less seriously!

Perspective

There is a very cheerful doorperson who works in my office building. She is always smiling, and whenever someone asks her how she is doing, she always replies, "I am awesome!" This afternoon while leaving my office, I heard the usual exchange again. This time, it was accompanied by an explanation.

Visitor: "How is your day going?"

Doorperson: "I am awesome!"

Visitor: "What makes your day awesome?"

Doorperson: "Perspective. I know it can always be worse!"

As I walked by, I had to smile to myself at the simple wisdom of this exchange. As long as you have perspective, you do not really need anything external to make your day awesome. You do not really need anything other than your outlook. You just have to look at it in a different way. As much as I am not a big fan of "it can always be worse," if it works to shift perspective in a positive direction, then that is what we are after here. Anxiety will often throw at you a singular way of looking at what is happening. That is surely not the only version! You can find a better version and you can create it!

The next time you feel challenged in your struggle with anxiety or you have a setback, ask yourself: "Is there another way to look at this situation/comment/outcome?" There often is. You can pick your perspective. You can choose a different story. You, and only you, get to decide this!

CHAPTER XVI.

Making Habits Stick!

"Change might not be fast and it isn't always easy. But with time and effort almost any habit can be reshaped."
—Charles Duhigg

"Forget safety. Live where you fear to live." —Rumi

Making anxiety management a habit requires time, patience, and perseverance.

What we know about building a habit is that it really takes practice to become better. I recommend scheduling a time daily to work on your anxiety skills – this can be as little as ten minutes a day. Once you have practiced a skill for twenty-one days, feel free to move on to a different skill while continuing to use the skill you have practiced as needed.

Making it stick may take more than twenty-one days. What the phrase "making it stick" means to me is that you are so well-practiced in using the skill that it becomes automatic, and when you do not practice it, you "miss" it and want to return to it. This may take months or years to establish – we are talking about life long habits – therefore in my opinion, they are well worth it.

Keeping Yourself Motivated

1. Keep It Positive

To keep yourself motivated, you can go two routes. You can beat yourself into submission, so to speak, by being your own harshest critic and making threats to yourself, or you can keep it positive. I meet with clients regularly who use negative self-motivation in various spheres of their life. In my experience, this is a surefire way to derail your progress and to feel lousy about any positive changes that you have made. Research has also shown that using negative self-motivation results in shorter duration of progress and more setbacks in goal attainment. In essence, you are less likely to stick with it or to keep working at it if you use criticism and harsh judgment to motivate yourself.

The positive approach allows you to use self-compassion, both when things are going well and you are reminding yourself to practice what you have learned, and when you experience a setback. If this is particularly difficult for you, as it is for many people, try speaking to yourself as you would to a good friend. Forgive yourself for past mistakes or times when you did not yet have the skills you have and are developing now. Forgive yourself for missed opportunities and past struggles. You can make changes only in the present, and that is the only fair request you can have of yourself. Start practicing the changes and new habits today and make it a life-long practice!

2. **Imagine the Possibilities**

It is important to imagine what you hope to achieve by working to manage your anxiety. To help with that vision, I suggest that you engage in the following exercise.

Write a letter to your future self. Keep this letter positive and forward-oriented.

Below is an example:

Dear Future Self,

I am excited to write this letter to you. It has been six months since you have committed to working on your panic and anxiety and I am seeing so many positive changes in you already! You are no longer afraid of panic. You are no longer limiting your activities based on whether or not you will experience panic or anxiety. Moreover, you have started taking more risks in your personal and professional life. You joined a civic organization and started participating in your neighborhood sports league. I know that you have started dating an interesting and attractive woman. I also know that you have been sharing your ideas at work much more openly and have asked your employer for more responsibility. As a result, you are currently working on several new projects.

I am really proud of you for all of the changes that you have been making! I imagine this is just the beginning. I know that it took a lot of guts to go on this journey, and I cannot wait to see where you will go in the next six months!
Love,
Your Past Self.

After you write this letter, please file it away and put a reminder on your calendar six months from now to open it. Then, go ahead and implement your action plan. Open the letter in six months – you have earned it! Read it and notice how you feel.

3. **Set Aside Time**
    We create our priorities these days based on how we spend our time. We are an increasingly time-poor society – there are just too many things vying for our limited time and attention. The only way to make any change a priority is to set aside a time

for it. By setting aside time, I do not mean that it will take a spot on your to-do list. I mean that you sit down and find a place for it on your calendar, regularly. You will treat this time like a sacred covenant with yourself, an important appointment that you will honor and devote your time and attention to on a regular basis.

4. **Create Accountability**

One of the most important things you can do to ensure your progress is to create a system of accountability. You can have a friend or loved one set aside time to chat with you about your goals or tasks on a regular basis. If you go this route, I recommend that you choose a friend or family member who is firm but delivers their feedback compassionately. They also need to be able to tell you frankly when you are not stepping up to the plate regarding the goals that you have committed to. Decide when you will have contact with them, and make sure it is scheduled on your calendar, like an appointment that you both commit to.

Another option is to retain the services of a licensed therapist who specializes in anxiety treatment. Here are some factors that you may wish to consider when selecting a therapist.

1. Training

    Be sure to ask whether the therapist has specialized training in treating anxiety disorders. Specifically, you want to find a therapist who has been trained to do Cognitive Behavioral Therapy (CBT) for Anxiety and who does Exposure Therapy as part of CBT. Cognitive Behavioral Therapy helps you address both thinking patterns and behaviors that make anxiety worse. This type of therapy helps you to address the mind game as well as face your fears with behavioral exposures or experiments. Exposure Therapy helps you face your fears by developing and implementing behavioral experiments that help challenge you to gradually face your feared symptoms or situations. The type of therapy is more important than where the therapist studied. These therapies have been research validated to have the most successful outcomes when it comes to treating anxiety.

2. Experience

    It is important that in addition to having specialized training, your therapist also has a good experience base in treating anxiety. Ask the therapist what portion of their practice is devoted to anxiety treatment. Experience base matters more than years in practice here. You are looking for someone whose practice is at least 50% devoted to clients who struggle with anxiety.

3. Connection

You need to pick a therapist who you feel understands anxiety and who speaks about it in a way that you understand. The therapist should be able to explain to you what therapy with them will be like and how you will be getting better. You should feel that their explanation makes sense and that there is a connection between the two of you. Trust your gut here. If it is not a fit, please move on. You will be discussing matters of an important and private nature, and you deserve to do that with someone you are comfortable with.

5 Tips for Making Habits Stick

1. First, repetition is key to forming habits. For example, if you would like to start going to the gym, plan to do it at the same time each week and you will be on your way to forming a positive habit.

2. Preplan for temptations that make you revert to old habits. If you plan on going to the gym on

Sunday mornings instead of catching up on the latest TV episodes you've missed, then you will want to tell yourself, "Instead of watching TV, I will go to the gym Sunday morning" to help in building that new healthy habit.

3. Adopt a "get back on track" mindset. We all slip up; rather than berating yourself, try to get back on track as soon as possible.

4. Do not rely purely on self-control. Rather than relying on self-control, find ways to help structure your surroundings to promote keeping that new healthy habit. If you are trying to eat healthier, you are better off not having that bag of chips at home; instead keep healthier snacks such as fruit visible and within reach – your mom had the right idea with putting that fruit basket on the kitchen counter! Having pre-made healthy snacks on hand and making your food ahead of time are all tricks that help promote your new habit.

5. Reward yourself for working hard! Plan a reward that does not compete with your goal. If your goal is to eat less sugary treats, then rather than

rewarding yourself with a cupcake, get a nice new tea mug for that herbal tea you drink when sugar cravings hit.

CHAPTER XVII

Relapse Prevention

"Success is not final, failure is not fatal: it is the courage to continue that counts." —*Winston S. Churchill*

"Life shrinks or expands in proportion to one's courage." —*Anais Nin*

Relapse prevention is a life-long habit. There are no short-cuts when it comes to your health. If you would like to have a healthy and fit body, you have to practice the habits of good nutrition and exercise consistently. Managing your mental health is no different. Practicing realistic, positive thinking styles as well as incorporating certain lifestyle habits and nixing others are essential to lifelong management of panic and anxiety.

Your Thoughts
Adopting a realistic but positive outlook on life has been studied extensively in the last few decades. The upshot is

that developing and maintaining an optimistic outlook aids in positive mental health maintenance and, in my opinion, in anxiety management. I add the word realistic because optimism is not a way to avoid or ignore your problems. It is simply being able to acknowledge what is, accepting your role and responsibility in it, and taking the most optimistic stance possible. Adopting a positive attitude does not mean that you just substitute positive thoughts in place of negative thoughts and hope that you believe them – your intelligent brain will not allow it! It means walking yourself through a realistic and positive scenario that you mostly believe has a chance of happening. I say "mostly" because we all have to act on faith from time to time. There is no absolute certainty – and so it is not necessary to require it of yourself here either!

Let's say, for instance, that you have just been laid off work. Realistic positive self-talk will sound something like this:

> I just lost my job. I have to revise my family bud-
> get and start looking for work. I will reach out to
> the colleagues in my field for any job opportuni-
> ties in order to get started. I will speak with my
> wife tonight to come up with a plan. Money will
> be tight for a while until I land another job, but I
> think that with some effort and persistence I will
> be able to find another job fairly soon. Until then,

I just have to focus on my strengths and create and follow a plan of action.

If you have just ended a romantic relationship, realistic positive talk sounds like this:

I am sad that my relationship with Sam just ended. I really thought that we had a future together, but it looks like we wanted different things and it made sense for us to part. Although it hurts now, I am sure that when I am ready, I will meet someone else who wants the same things out of life as I do: marriage, children, and a house in the country. Until then, I need some time to heal and be with friends so I can be ready to date in the near future.

Practicing Your Skills

The only way to keep your skills sharp is to practice them. For this reason, we look at any anxiety-provoking situation as simply an opportunity to practice your skills. The same is true for any panic symptoms you may experience. Anxiety loves comfort and safety. By now you know that I call this avoidance, and that avoidance creates more anxiety. It is therefore my position that if you are someone who struggles with anxiety, a "comfortable" life is your enemy, and you must intentionally and consistently seek out opportunities to take appropriate risks in your life. Comfortable, in this instance, means a life that is very predictable and routinized with few risks taken by you, a life where the "status quo" is a mask for stagnation and avoidance. What taking risks means for you is unique to you and your circumstances. Everyone's idea of risk is different, and some risks may be appropriate for one person but not another.

- If you are afraid of public speaking, seek out opportunities to give a toast at a wedding, do a presentation at work, or speak up at your community meeting. You may even consider joining a speaking organization such as Toastmasters.

- If you are a homebody, find a way to venture away from home and travel as far as time and money allows. Start by exploring new places close to home, and then venture farther and farther out. Create your own explorations and adventures.

- If you do not like crowded places, start introducing yourself to larger and larger gatherings, starting from house parties to street festivals, and move on to large shopping malls.

- If you are afraid of being ridiculed, seek out opportunities to share your opinion: join a book club,

find a civic organization and volunteer for a leader-
ship role, speak up at work and social functions.

- If you are afraid of making mistakes, find opportunities to learn a new skill such as dancing, a sport
with which you are not familiar, or a new hobby.
This will provide the many mistake-making opportunities you need as you are learning something
that is new and unfamiliar to you.

How do we know when it is a good time to do this?
Anytime you feel too comfortable and experience an
absence of anxiety in your life, it likely means you are
lacking in anxiety-busting practice. Although almost
everyone who has struggled with anxiety wishes for its
absence entirely, anxiety is necessary and beneficial to
us. Feeling too safe is sometimes the very thing that per-
petuates it. So let's get some practice and take some life-
enriching risks!

Everyday Anxiety Management

So your anxiety starts to come up. On a scale of one to
ten, it is only a three, but you start fidgeting, running
through the "what-ifs" in your mind and wondering if
you will ever be the sort of person to just roll with the
punches and not fret about things. You wonder if things
will get worse, if you will ever feel normal, and whether
if or when you have children, they too will be anxious

just like you. In that moment, anxiety has won. It has taken you out of your current reality and projected you into some undesirable future scenario – but it does not have to.

Managing anxiety starts with acknowledging that the only changes we have the power to make are in the present. It means accepting that we do not control the future or other people's opinions. It means living with the stance that no matter what we have done in the past, we always have that next moment in life to act differently.

Start by regularly rating your anxiety without judgment on a scale of one to ten, three times a day. You may wish to combine this with a routine you already have, such as breakfast, lunch, and dinner. Notice the number and resist the urge to judge it. Your entire task consists of developing awareness around what a particular rating of anxiety feels like in your body. *This is a three. Okay. This is a five. Okay, got it! This is a seven – seems familiar.* That is all. Just notice the level of anxiety. Take away the comparisons, the judgments, and the bad recollections of anxieties past.

Next, listen for your inner voice. Is it taking you down the road of anxiety and feeding you thinking errors? Are you looking at the negatives, wondering about terrible future scenarios, dismissing your own strengths? Notice this and change course as needed. Remember, you do not have to believe everything that anxiety tells you or wants you to believe. You do not have to respond as though it is danger when it is just discomfort.

Are unhelpful beliefs getting activated? Respond with reaffirming helpful beliefs, and do not judge yourself for the slip ups. You are only human, and you will make mistakes. After all, slip ups are just opportunities to practice your skills. The good news is that you do not have to stay there – you can get back on track!

Are you avoiding people, places, or situations in order to manage your anxiety? If so, it is time to start re-engaging. Create a list of people, places, and situations you have been avoiding, rate each item from lowest to highest on the anxiety level it produces, and start with the lowest item on the list. Proceed on to the next item until you have completed your list. If you find this step difficult, you may want to enlist a support person or an anxiety therapist to help you.

Finally, look at what it means for you to be living a life that is fulfilling and full of meaning. Is your life peopled with caring family and friends? Do you have the intellectual stimulation you need? Do you feel connected to the community and the world in a way that gives you meaning? Is there room for fun, relaxation, and playfulness? Think about these questions, and if it feels like one or more of these areas needs your attention, give it some reflection and write down one action step you can take to make it more of a priority in your life.

Practicing Discomfort

Anxiety loves and flourishes in comfort. Since most of us enjoy feeling comfortable, this becomes a challenge. Your symptoms may resolve, and if you look at that as an opportunity to rest and settle into a comfortable pattern, that is typically when anxiety rears its ugly head. The solution is to seek out our comfort zones, and to stretch further than they expand.

So wait a minute, you have done all this work and made all these changes so that you can feel more comfortable, and here I am telling you to seek out discomfort? YES! If it sounds counterintuitive – it is! It also helps with relapse prevention. We are constantly growing and evolving. If we are not, we are probably avoiding some necessary risks. Avoidance breeds anxiety. Comfort breeds anxiety. Safety breeds anxiety. Wishing to be cocooned in safety and comfort breeds more anxiety. So… YES! In order to beat anxiety, we need to seek out those opportunities for discomfort in order to maintain our gains. In my opinion, we need to make it our ongoing mission!

CHAPTER XVIII.

Are You All In?

"The most authentic thing about us is our capacity to create, to overcome, to endure, to transform, to love and to be greater than our suffering." — *Ben Okri*

I was at a conference recently, where Shawn Shepard, an inspirational speaker, listed a few criteria for reaching your goals:

1. Openness

2. Asking the Right Questions

3. Being All In

"Being All In." That was the difference between people who reached their goals and those who did not. Being all in – that can be a little scary. We like to protect ourselves. We protect ourselves from loss. We protect ourselves from disappointment. We are a safety conscious species – particularly so when we are anxious. We are skeptical and we are reserved in our approach. We make contingency plans, we do not put all our eggs into one basket, and we do not Go All In!

It felt like a riddle to me. Paradoxical though it was, it also felt like that is what we most need to do. We cannot let go of our old thinking unless we go all in. We cannot commit to a new habit if we are married to a previous one. We cannot really say we gave it a fair shot if we did not go all in. And yet, I get it – it is scary. I get it – we have a need to be vulnerable and a competing need to protect ourselves. I will invite you to go all in anyway.

Here is my proposed pathway for going all in when you believe it is the right thing to do, but you feel scared:

1. Ask yourself: what is the alternative?

   What is the alternative to not going all in? Really look at whether you are willing to do it. If you broke your legs and could not walk without intensive physical therapy would you decide to only sometimes practice the exercises? Or would you go all in? If you stay like this and do not take steps to resolve your anxiety, how will you feel in a week? A month? A year? Five years from now? Let your answers be your guide.

2. Predict and prune the negative brain chatter.

   The anxious brain is very good at generating anxious mind chatter, for example:

"What is this does not work?"

"What if I cannot beat my anxiety or panic?"

"What if there is another book I should read before I try the strategies in this one?"

It is vital that you are able to predict that right before you embark on any goal, your anxiety about that goal may become heightened, and that this negative mind chatter is to be expected. The good news is that you do not have to treat each thought as equally important. Decide not to indulge the what-ifs and focus only on what is – limit your focus to what you need and what needs to be done rather than what can go wrong.

3. Let the data, not your fear, be your guide.

Yes – you read that right, I said let data be your guide! We have emotional and experiential data. We can use rating scales to see if our anxiety is trending down. We can use data to see how long it takes us to recover from a panic attack and whether that time is getting shorter. We can use this data in the face of fear to gauge our progress. And if that is true then there is no barrier to going all in – all we have to do is allow the data to be our guide.

4. Make a decision to stick it out for a fair trial.

Earlier on in the book I shared my experience with trying to read many books about anxiety very quickly in an attempt to find a solution. This did not yield positive results, and so I do not recommend it. I often see this phenomenon in new parents – they get five different books on taking care of a baby and then try to use all of the advice with the intention of being comprehensive in their approach. More often than not, this backfires. By pulling bits and pieces from different systems, we often end up with contradictory advice. At best, it is confusing and frustrating. At worst, it plainly does not work, because the different pieces of these systems just do not work well together. An approach that works better is to try one system at a time, decide to implement its strategies, and gather data over time to determine how well it is working for you.

If you are still hesitant, it helps to ask yourself the following question; "What is the worst that can happen if I try to overcome my anxiety?" Usually the answer is, "The worst thing that can happen is that nothing changes." That is usually the answer when we take a chance. We may be disappointed, but we are no worse off for trying.

The next question is, "What is the best thing that can happen?" The answer may be something like, "The best thing that can happen is that I learn to overcome my anxiety and panic," or "The best thing that can happen is that I reduce or eliminate my anxiety, so that I can live my life with more freedom!" Which one of those sounds more compelling to you? If it is the second one, go ahead – Be All In – you are no worse off for trying and you have everything to gain!

CHAPTER XIX

Anxiety Management in the Real World

"Don't be afraid to take a big step if one is indicated; you can't cross a chasm in two small jumps."
—David Lloyd George

You've come this far, and you may be wondering what's next. My hope for you is that you continue to manage your anxiety. My experience is that in the real world the opportunities to practice your skills occur regularly and are wholly unplanned and abundant. This is good news, if you are able to see it as such. In my practice I will often see someone a few months after they have stopped therapy for a "tune-up" session. Frequently, the puzzling question during that session is, "sometimes it still feels like I am about to have that old feeling – and I wonder, am I going to backtrack?" This is an important question. I like to look at it from the standpoint of whether any single feeling is an indication of progress; in my view they are not. It is simply a reminder about how far you have come. Let me explain; you may experience some anxiety and anxious sensations throughout your life – this is human and is not a cause for concern. What is important is whether or not these sensations create a downward spiral of negativity, worry about the future, and foreboding disaster. If they do not – you are in good shape.

Move past the "What If?"

Recently, a client in my consultation room was lamenting that even with all of the progress he has made working through considerable panic and social anxiety, he still has moments that feel like everything is about to collapse. I asked him what he does with those moments, and as we talked it became clear that while he occasionally experienced some anxious discomfort, he persevered and did not let it stop him. He was taking more risks in his career, and this naturally involved facing some novel situations and more public speaking opportunities, which created a sense of uncertainty and increased anxious feelings. However, he noticed that these moments did not last and did not plague him, and that by and large he was managing them successfully. He was able to do this because he was taking action. In the real world, just like in the world of doing anxiety exposures, relief is on the other side of action. When you find yourself pondering whether you can do something that makes you anxious, I encourage you to think about how you can do it instead of if you can do it.

Sometimes You Need a Hard Reset

At times, we feel rushed, tense, and depleted of energy, and we do not know why. Sometimes it is our life that's the problem. We hurry, we are busy, we take on projects, the kids get sick, and there is no time for us. During those times I encourage you to step back and do a "hard reset." Just as our smartphones, tablets, and computers periodically need time to power down and reconfigure, so do we. We need that time to reassess, to readjust and to plan ahead. Sometimes that time means we need to take care of our physical needs, get more sleep, exercise, or take care of a medical issue. At other times it means attending to our spiritual, creative, or relationship needs. This often means slowing down and asking yourself: "What do I most need right now?" Listen to that answer, however quietly it appears. Discard the urge to dismiss that answer as unimportant or self-indulgent. When you greet that answer head on, without judgment, and focus on how you can have more of what you need, you are on your way to feeling less anxious. If you cannot get all of what you need, set up a timeline for when you can get some of what you need and how you can keep yourself on track to your goals. For example, you can tell a friend, therapist, or significant other about your goals, set reminders on your calendar to reassess, or track goals in a personal journal.

Rewrite Your Rulebook

Up until now your rulebook has been heavily influenced by anxiety. I would venture that it has also contributed heavily to promoting and increasing your anxiety. Anxiety has you live by a certain code; if you deviate from that code, there is a price to pay – which is usually self-deprecation, shame, and doubt. In the real world, we all come into situations where our performance is less than stellar, we are embarrassed, or our flaws are made publicly visible.

This is the stuff most frightening nightmares are made of, therefore we are most likely to follow rules that try to prevent these scenarios from happening. The problem with these rules, other than they are simply ineffective at preventing all possible negative outcomes, is that they take us very far away from being able to engage in our life and relationships. Recently, a client lamented how hard social situations were for her, because try as she might to control her own behavior, other people simply did not follow the same set of rules, which made interactions with friends and family a source of great anxiety. After all, our internal beliefs and feelings may tell us that people close to us might also follow a strict set of rules, because negative attention and therefore embarrassment are just around the corner. As you might imagine, I told my client she needed to get rid of the rule book, which led to a perplexed look – followed by loud laughter. Yes – laughter! Tossing your rulebook is a celebration of freedom.

Create a Safe Universe Belief

We live in a world where painful and sometimes scary and tragic things happen. Of course, many wonderful things happen as well; new life brought into the world, love, kindness, community, and laughter are also abundant. In the face of such juxtapositions, we are faced with a choice. Do we believe that this universe is by and large dangerous, malicious, and hollow, or do we believe that this universe is safe, benevolent, and abundant? Anxiety has a clear preference for the former, which leads to trepidation and avoidance, which in turn lead to refusing challenges and fearing that the next disaster is just around the corner. When we look at our world as scary, it becomes so; we notice only the danger signals, and we then take in this information and use it to confirm our bias. Similarly, if we look at this world as safe, we start seeing proof of it being the safe place we hope it is. I find it immensely easier to live in a world where the only dangers we need to deal with are the ones that cross our path, a world that allows us to be free of all the hypothetical dangers we may encounter.

Allow yourself to believe that this world is a safe and secure place.

Books about Anxiety, Worry and Panic

Anxiety Free: Unravel Your Fears Before They Unravel You,
Robert L. Leahy, PhD

Don't Panic: Taking Control of Anxiety Attacks,
Reid Wilson

Feel the Fear and Do It Anyway, Susan Jeffers, PhD

Hope and Help for Your Nerves, Claire Weekes, MD
Overcoming Social Anxiety: Step by Step, Thomas A.
Richards, PD et al.

*Quiet: The Power of Introverts in a World That Can't
Stop Talking,* Susan Cain

The Anxiety and Phobia Workbook, Edmond Bourne, PhD

*The Cognitive Behavioral Workbook for Anxiety: A Step By
Step Program,* William J. Knauss, EdD and
Jon Carlson, PsyD

*The Mindfulness and Acceptance Workbook for Anxiety:
A Guide to Breaking Free from Anxiety, Phobias, and
Worry Using Acceptance and Commitment Therapy,*
John P. Forsyth, PhD and Georg H. Eifert, PhD

The Mindfulness and Acceptance Workbook for Social Anxiety and Shyness: Using Acceptance and Commitment Therapy to Free Yourself from Fear and Reclaim Your Life, Jan E. Fleming, Nancy L. Kocovski, and Zindel V. Segal

The Relaxation and Stress Reduction Workbook, Martha Davis, Elizabeth Robbins Eshelman and Matthew McKay

The Shyness & Social Anxiety Workbook: Proven Techniques for Overcoming Your Fears, Martin M. Antony and Richard P. Swinson

The Worry Trick: How Your Brain Tricks You Into Expecting the Worst and What to Do, David Carbonell, PhD

Thriving with Social Anxiety: Daily Strategies for Overcoming Anxiety and Building Self-Confidence, Hattie C. Cooper and Kyle MacDonald

When Panic Attacks, David D. Burns, MD

Anxiety Books for Teens

101 Ways to Conquer Teen Anxiety: Simple Tips, Techniques and Strategies for Overcoming Anxiety, Worry and Panic, Dr. Thomas McDonagh and Jon Patrick Hatcher

A Still Quiet Place for Teens: A Mindfulness Workbook to Ease Stress and Difficult Emotions, Amy Saltzman, MD

Anxiety Sucks! A Teen Survival Guide (Volume 1), Natasha Daniels, LCSW

How to Like Yourself: A Teen's Guide to Quieting Your Inner Critic and Building Lasting Self Esteem, Cheryl M. Bradshaw

Mindfulness for Teen Anxiety: A Workbook for Overcoming Teen Anxiety at Home, at School, and Everywhere Else, Christopher Willard, PsyD

My Anxious Mind: A Teen's Guide to Managing Anxiety and Panic, Michael M. Tompkins, Katherine A. Martinez and Michael Sloan

Not by Chance, How Parents can Boost Their Teen's Success In and After Treatment, Tim R. Thayne, PhD

The Anxiety Survival Guide for Teens: CBT Skills to Overcome Fear, Worry and Panic, Jennifer Shannon LMFT

The Anxiety Workbook for Teens: Activities to Help You Deal with Anxiety and Worry, Lisa M. Schab, LCSW

The Panic Workbook for Teens: Breaking the Cycle of Fear, Worry, and Panic Attacks, Debra Kissen, PhD and Bari Goldman Cohen, PhD

The Perfectionism Workbook for Teens: Activities to Help You Reduce Anxiety and Get Things Done, Ann Marie Dobosz, MA

The Shyness and Social Anxiety Workbook for Teens: CBT and ACT Skills to Help You Build Social Confidence, Jennifer Shannon, LMFT and Doug Shannon

Anxiety Books for Kids

12 Annoying Monsters: Self-talk for Kids with Anxiety,
Dawn Meredith

*Anxious Kids, Anxious Parents: 7 Ways to Stop the Worry
Cycle and Raise Courageous and Independent Children*,
Reid Wilson, PhD

*Freeing Your Child from Anxiety: Powerful, Practical
Solutions to Overcome Your Child's Fears, Worries, and
Phobias*, Tama L. Chansky

*Growing Up Brave: Expert Strategies for Helping Your Child
Overcome Fear, Stress, and Anxiety*, Donna B. Pincus

*Helping Your Anxious Child: A Step-by-Step Guide for
Parents*, Ronald Rapee, PhD and Ann Wignall, D Psych

*Master of Mindfulness: How to Be Your Own Superhero in
Times of Stress*, Laurie Grossman and Mr. Musumeci's 5th
Grade Class

Playing with Anxiety: Casey's Guide for Teens and Kids,
Reid Wilson, PhD

Please Explain Anxiety to Me! Simple Biology and Solutions for Children and Parents, Laurie E. Zelinger and Jordan Zelinger

The Anxiety Cure for Kids: A Guide for Parents and Children, Elizabeth DuPont Spencer, Robert L. DuPont and Caroline DuPont

The Girl Who Never Made Mistakes, Mark Pett and Gary Rubinstein

The Relaxation and Stress Reduction Workbook for Kids: Help for Children to Cope with Stress, Anxiety and Transitions, Lawrence Shapiro, PhD and Robin Sprague

What to Do When You're Scared and Worried: A Guide for Kids, James J. Crist

What to Do When You Worry Too Much: A Kid's Guide to Overcoming Anxiety, Dawn Huebner and Bonnie Matthews

Why Smart Kids Worry and What Parents Can Do to Help, Allison Edwards

Wilma Jeanne the Worry Machine, Julia Cook and Anita DuFalla

Books for Those Whose Loved One is Struggling

How You Can Survive When They're Depressed: Living and Coping with Depression Fallout, Anne Sheffield, Mike Wallace, Donald F. Klein

Loving Someone with Anxiety: Understanding and Helping Your Partner, Kate N. Thieda

Talking to Anxiety: Simple Ways to Support Someone in Your Life Who Suffers From Anxiety, Claudia J. Strauss

Talking to Depression: Simple Ways to Connect When Someone in Your Life is Depressed, Claudia J. Strauss

Additional Resources

Anxiety and Depression Association of America
www.adaa.org
8701 Georgia Ave., Suite #412
Silver Spring, MD 20910
(240) 485-1001

Anxiety Disorders Association of Canada
http://www.anxietycanada.ca

Anxiety UK
www.anxietyuk.org.uk
08444 775 774

Fear of Flying
http://www.fearofflying.com/

International OCD foundation
https://iocdf.org
International OCD Foundation, Inc.
P.O. Box 961029
Boston, MA 02196
(617) 973-5801

Mindfulness — UCLA Mindfulness Research Center
Free Guided Meditation Recordings
http://marc.ucla.edu/body.cfm?id=22

National Sleep Foundation
https://sleepfoundation.org

Worry and Anxiety in Children
www.worrywisekids.org

Acknowledgements

I owe a debt of gratitude to the many people who supported me in the writing and publishing process. To Brenda Knight and the team at Mango Publishing, you were enthusiastic about this project from the start. Thank you for your seamless introduction into the world of publishing and all of your help throughout the editing and publishing process.

To my loving parents, thank you for your love and support always.

To my daughter, Maya, for your laughter.

To John G. Duffy, thank you for your guidance, mentorship and feedback into this work from its inception.

To my clients, I am forever your student and I learn more about fearlessness and anxiety busting from you than from anyone else.

To my husband Alex, you make all of this possible through your encouragement and humor. Thank you for your support through this and all my other adventures.

About the Author

Dr. Helen Odessky is a Chicago-based Licensed Clinical Psychologist, speaker, coach and anxiety expert. She has been working with individuals, teens, and couples for nearly 15 years. She is a highly sought-after public speaker and regularly speaks to corporate clients through her speaker's bureau work. Dr. Odessky regularly blogs on anxiety and communicates regularly with her growing base of followers on Facebook and Twitter. You can learn more about her at: www.yourchicagotherapist.com